DIABETES 101

REVISED AND EXPANDED
2ND EDITION

A Pure and Simple Guide for People Who Use Insulin

BETTY PAGE BRACKENRIDGE, M.S., R.D., C.D.E.,
AND RICHARD O. DOLINAR, M.D.

Library of Congress Cataloging-in-Publication Data

Brackenridge, Betty Page
Diabetes 101: A pure and simple guide
for people who use insulin.

1. Diabetes--Popular works. (1. Diabetes.)
I. Dolinar, Richard O. II. Title
RC660.4.D65 1993 616.4'62 89-37754
ISBN 1-56561-024-5

Edited by Donna Hoel
Production Manager: Claire Lewis
Printed in the United States of America

Published by
CHRONIMED Publishing
P.O. Box 47945
Minneapolis, MN 55447-9727

Before You Begin

A lot of information is available to the person with diabetes. There are mountains of pamphlets, instruction sheets, and diet forms. There are rooms filled with films, slides, and tapes. There is a stream of committed health professionals gushing sometimes mind-numbing torrents of well-meaning words. And there are many books.

So why write another one? Great question. And we think we have a great answer. We wrote this little book because there is a need.

Not a need for another *War and Peace* of diabetes. A need, rather, for a brief and readable guide to important basic information needed every day by people who take insulin to control their diabetes.

Some information about diabetes is vital to daily living. That information is in this book. Some additional liberating information about diabetes is also included.

But some things are NOT in this book because everything just can't be learned all at once. A lot of information about diabetes that is interesting—especially to doctors and nurses—but not necessary for daily diabetes care has been left out. And certain advanced skills have also been omitted. There are wonderful books that cover such topics in great detail. We encourage you to read them when you have the need. Today, though, read this little book.

We've been told it's helpful.

Betty Brackenridge
Richard Dolinar

Acknowledgments

This book carries the names of only two authors. In reality, many others have contributed greatly to its development and we thank them all for their help and encouragement. Our primary thanks must go to our patients. They have taught us about the reality of living with diabetes and, in that way, have shown us the difference between what they truly *needed* to know and what we *thought* they should know.

Dr. Dolinar extends special thanks to the outstanding group of physicians present at Duke University Medical Center in the early 1980s who had a major impact on his interest in and approach to diabetes. They include Harold Lebovitz, M.D., head of the Department of Endocrinology at that time; George Eisenbarth, M.D., Ph.D., who provided many unique insights regarding Type I diabetes; George "Jay" Ellis, M.D., who emphasized the importance of practical patient education and who modeled a dynamic problem-solving method of diabetes management, and Warner Burch, M.D., who contributed his practical approach to patient care. Harry McPherson, M.D., Frank Neelon, M.D., Jerome Feldman, M.D., Charles Johnson, M.D., Mark Feinglos, M.D., Marc Drezner, M.D., and Titus Allen, M.D., were very kind to share their many clinical "pearls of wisdom." And thanks also to Mrs. Johnnie Alexander who provided unique support in her own very special way.

Betty Brackenridge warmly acknowledges the many colleagues who have contributed to *Diabetes 101* with their skillful advice and exceptional example, especially Keith Campbell, Cathy Feste, Bob Anderson, Christine Tobin, and Hope Warshaw. She also wishes to acknowledge the members of the American Association of Diabetes Educators who dedicate their love and skill to opening windows of freedom for those with diabetes.

Dedication

This second edition of *Diabetes 101* is dedicated with deep love and thanks to our parents—those who are gone and those who are still with us.

Albert and Antoinette Dolinar

J.D. and Elizabeth Page

SPECIAL NOTE: Consult your doctor before making any change in your diabetes care plan. The information contained in this book can help you become more involved and informed regarding your diabetes management. But it is NOT a substitute for regular diabetes care by your physician or for personalized diabetes education.

Table of Contents

Section One: The Basics

Section Two: The Flashy Plays

Helpful Tables and Charts

Section One

The Basics

1

The Journey:
Introduction

Clowns to the left of me,
Jokers to the right.
Here I am, stuck in the middle with you.
                                        —Steelers Wheel

Not long ago, in a place not far from where you live, a young man named Mike began a journey. On the surface, it seemed to be a simple quest. He was looking for a way to be healthy and live freely in his unique situation.

And he seemed well-equipped to find what he was looking for. He was bright, hard-driving, and ambitious. He devoted long hours to the work he loved, and he had the support of good friends and family.

But the quest was necessary because, in spite of his many gifts, he had a problem: He had diabetes. And it was getting in the way of nearly everything he wanted and needed to do.

Having diabetes meant getting up early enough every morning for an insulin shot, a blood sugar reading, and a good breakfast. No jumping out of bed at the last minute, skipping breakfast, and sprinting to the train for Mike.

Having diabetes also meant his day was sometimes interrupted by insulin reactions—periods of sweating and confusion brought on by a sudden drop in his blood sugar level. Once he had one while making an important pitch to the top management at work. He had to excuse himself to get something to eat. Now he worries that the boss may see him as weaker or less able than he once did.

And meals were another problem. Business lunches eaten on the run didn't have much in common with the advice the dietitian gave him when his diabetes was diagnosed.

But lunches were a snap compared with dinner meetings with prolonged "happy hours." Discussing business over drinks could delay a meal for hours. How much could he drink? When should he take his insulin? What's more, the dinners often took place in fine restaurants where the menus offered rich meals and gooey desserts—not the best fare for someone concerned about health.

The list of frustrations seemed endless, but Mike was determined to find a way to take diabetes off the front burner. He was sure his life would get back to normal if only he could keep the diabetes "pot" from always being at a full boil.

His doctor took a different view. He often seemed to blame Mike for the wildly swinging blood sugars. He implied, insinuated, and at times even openly accused the young man of "cheating." But sometimes the blood sugars were too high even when Mike had followed his diabetes plan to the letter. The doctor just wouldn't believe him.

In fact, most of the time, the doctor acted as if Mike's life was getting in the way of his diabetes, rather than the other way around. And so his quest for a better life began with the search for a new doctor.

His first attempt was with one who seemed to solve all of the problems on the very first visit. With a slight smile and a comforting pat on the shoulder, the doctor told Mike to stop worrying so much about his blood sugar.

"That's my job, Mike," he said. "Just take your insulin every day, and I'll take care of everything else."

This seemed like the answer to Mike's prayers. It certainly was easier. What a relief not to be constantly worried about his blood sugar. But it wasn't long before he noticed that his energy level was falling and that he was losing weight without trying.

It was a familiar feeling. It was just the way he'd felt when he first developed diabetes. He was just 16 at the time. He remembered losing weight for several weeks while he grew weaker and weaker. He'd had a terrible thirst that never seemed to go away, no matter how much he drank.

His parents took him to the family doctor in his old home town. The doctor was the one to give Mike the unwelcome news that he had diabetes. He told him that his blood sugar was almost 400. The doctor explained that all of Mike's symptoms were being caused by that high blood sugar level. He said that when too much sugar gets into the blood, some spills over into the urine, just like water spills over a dam. More and more water is needed to carry away the extra sugar. Losing all of that water produces the terrible thirst that Mike remembered so well.

The sugar being lost in the urine was full of calories—food energy. And that was where the weight loss was coming from. Energy from some of the food he was eating never got used by his body. Instead, it flowed out in the sugary urine produced by his high blood sugar level. It was just as if he'd never eaten that food—and so he lost weight.

One night, when he was thinking about how tired he felt, he noticed an item in a diabetes magazine. "A growing body of evidence strongly suggests that the long-term complications of diabetes may be prevented or delayed by excellent control of the blood glucose level," the article proclaimed. Mike knew that his diabetes was out of control just by how awful he felt. And according to the article, he needed to get his blood sugar under control as soon as possible to decrease his chances of developing problems in the future. It was time to resume his journey.

His next stop brought him to a very enthusiastic physician. This doctor agreed that good blood sugar control could help limit the complications of diabetes. Unfortunately, though, he also viewed normal blood sugars as a sort of Holy Grail. He pursued them with a zeal that would have made any Crusader proud.

"Diabetes touches every part of your life, Mike. Everything that affects it has to be carefully managed. Do exactly as I say and I'll have you in control in no time."

Then the doctor took over, putting every detail of Mike's life on a schedule. Even occasional activities like a game of tennis were included on the timetable.

It seemed that every hour of the day held some task related to diabetes. Mike began scheduling fewer business appointments. He even canceled meetings entirely on some days in order to get it all done. He was supposed to weigh and measure everything he ate—an impossible task for someone who ate in restaurants nearly every day. But even more frustrating, the doctor's schedule was at odds with the times set for meals and coffee breaks at work.

Mike felt his sanity slipping away.

The last straw came when he returned to the doctor's office with his record book. It contained all of the blood sugar values he had carefully and painfully gathered since the last visit. But the doctor only gave the book a casual glance as he thumbed rapidly through the pages.

Tossing the record book aside, the doctor gazed sternly at the young man. "These blood sugars aren't good enough yet. We need to tighten up your schedule."

Mike's jaw dropped open in disbelief, but the doctor didn't even notice. He was too busy adding more blood sugar readings to the schedule.

"You'll have to get rid of these tennis games, too."

"But isn't exercise good for my diabetes?"

Without even acknowledging Mike's question, the doctor proceeded to "tighten the schedule," making even more extreme demands on the young man's time. When he finished, he turned and disappeared through the exam room door. Poof! He was gone.

Mike hadn't even had a chance to reply. He couldn't believe it!

Another appointment had ended and he still didn't have answers to his questions. He'd taken a half day off work. He'd struggled through traffic to get there on time. And then he'd cooled his heels in a waiting room full of magazines so old that they could have been unearthed in an archaeological dig. But in spite of all that, he'd had less than five minutes of the doctor's time and *none* of his attention. It was all too much. So was the bill.

It was time to leave . . . permanently.

And so Mike took up the search once again.

Many months, many doctors, and many dollars later, he finally found the doctor he was looking for. The rest of this book is the story of what Mike then learned that put him where he belonged—in control of both his life and his diabetes.

When you control diabetes, it won't control you.

2

Riding the Bicycle: An Overview

I get by with a little help from my friends,
Gonna try with a little help from my friends.
—The Beatles

One evening the search took Mike to a diabetes meeting at a local hospital. The woman sitting next to him seemed friendly enough, so he struck up a conversation. As they talked he realized that, even though she had diabetes and understood his problems, she wasn't having the same difficulties herself.

"Your doctors have been taking responsibility for your diabetes," she said. "That doesn't work. What you need is someone to teach you how to take control for yourself. Why don't you try my doctor?"

Since the woman seemed to be doing so well, Mike agreed to try just one more doctor. He called for an appointment.

A few days later, when he met the doctor for the first time, he blurted out his frustrations. "Doctor," he said, "I want to enjoy my life without thinking about diabetes every minute of the day. I want to work hard, have some fun, and travel. I want to have my old energy level back and to stay healthy. I want to be myself again. Is that too much to ask?"

"No, it's not, Mike. If we work together, I think we can do it."

"I'm glad to hear you say that, Doc. I was beginning to think I was in this all alone."

The doctor continued. "Do you remember when you were a kid and just learning to ride a bike? Managing your diabetes is like that. First of all, it takes time. You didn't jump on a two-wheeler and pedal away the first time. In the same way, it'll take you a while to master the skills that will put you in charge of your diabetes."

The doctor then pointed out, "Just like no one else could ride the bike for you, no one else can control diabetes for you either. That's why it's so important to master the skills yourself. It's up to you.

"Do you remember the great feeling you had when riding that bike got to be second nature? When you found you could ride it anywhere? So what if a cat ran in front of you or there were potholes in the road? You just made a few corrections and kept rolling right along. Eventually you probably even learned to do tricks on the bike like riding with no hands. What a great feeling, even though it gave your mom gray hairs and took years off of her life.

"The more you rode, the easier it became. Managing your diabetes will become much easier with practice, too. But first you need to learn the basics."

"What basics?" Mike wanted to know.

"Insulin, food, activity, and timing. Once you understand those, you can play to win. You'll get feedback from blood glucose monitoring. Then you'll use that information to make corrections in the timing or amounts of insulin, food, or exercise to produce even better control of your blood sugars.

"When you get that far, you'll be ready to deal with a few potholes in the road: delayed meals, eating in new places, getting sick, and so on. You'll learn to make the necessary corrections and just keep rolling along."

"You mean I'll be able to do all of that myself?"

"Yes, and, if you want, you can even learn to do the diabetes equivalent of 'trick' riding, like taking a European vacation or rafting down the Colorado River. We'll talk about that when you've developed a bit more skill.

"But your first job is to learn the basics."

Learning to control your diabetes

- Takes Effort
- Takes Time
- Takes Practice

BUT. . .

It's Worth It!

3

Keeping the Fire
Burning: Insulin

Come on baby, light my fire.
—Jim Morrison

"Regulating your blood sugar is like managing a fire in the
fireplace of a cabin in the woods," explained the doctor.
"That cabin is like a cell inside your body.

"Sugar in the blood is the fuel supply for your body's
energy-producing fire, just as the logs in the woodpile are
the fuel for the fire in the fireplace. Insulin keeps the cabin
door open so fuel can be brought in from the woodpile and
placed in the fireplace.

"Without insulin, the door closes, cutting off the fuel
supply. When that happens, your body's energy-produc-

ing fire can't burn as it should. That's why you *must* take your insulin every day, without fail. It's as basic to your survival as the food you eat, the water you drink, and the air you breathe."

The doctor went on to explain that insulin needs vary from person to person. Each insulin dose must be carefully tailored to fit those needs like a custom-made suit. And insulin needs will change a bit from day to day—just as you sometimes need to tighten the belt or loosen the collar button, even when a suit is basically a good fit. The "fit" of the insulin dose has to be adjusted slightly when high or low blood sugars tell us it's not quite right.

Mike felt uneasy about the prospect of adjusting his own insulin. That was something his doctors had always done for him.

"Don't worry," the doctor assured him. "We'll be doing this one step at a time. You'll learn exactly how to make small adjustments in your insulin doses using a method I call 'Dynamic Insulin Dosing^{SM}.' Your doctors have been using static dosing, which means they set your insulin doses at each office visit and the doses remained the same until your next appointment. Of course, that could be weeks or even months away."

Mike understood the drawbacks of static dosing firsthand. When his insulin dose was set too high, he had repeated low blood sugar reactions and was eating constantly to "feed" that extra insulin. He would feel awful, and his blood sugars would gradually go out of control.

At other times, when the dose the doctor set was too low, Mike would go for weeks with high blood sugars, waiting for his next appointment and the needed dose change. The high blood sugars made him feel tired and run down. Once again, his diabetes would be out of control.

The doctor continued, "Now that it's possible to take your blood sugar between office visits using a home blood glucose monitor, we don't have to settle for static dosing. We can use Dynamic Insulin Dosing."

"What's Dynamic Insulin Dosing, Doc?"

"It's a simple system you can use to adjust your own insulin doses between office visits. Today I'll make an estimate of your dose based on your current dose, your weight, and your blood sugars. But that will only be a starting point.

"Using your blood test results and the Dynamic Insulin Dosing Guidelines,"* you'll make stepwise adjustments in the doses to gradually improve your blood sugar control. You won't be wasting time waiting around for our next visit. You'll be able to fine-tune the insulin to meet your needs as time goes along. You'll be in charge."

"That makes sense. But it's so different from the way my other doctors have done it," Mike commented.

"It's going to be a big change for you, all right. But Dynamic Dosing will help us get much closer to the blood

* See page 23 for Dynamic Dosing Guidelines

sugar levels your body achieved on its own before you had diabetes. There's a fair amount of research showing good blood sugar control decreases your chances of developing the long-term complications of diabetes. So I want to offer you every possible tool to improve your diabetes control.

"One of those tools is Dynamic Dosing. We'll use it as we combine different types of insulin. You see, no one type of insulin can keep your blood sugar in control over a whole day. Sometimes you need a lot of insulin and sometimes you only need a little. You need more than one shot a day and more than one type of insulin to meet that changing demand. We'll use both a short-acting insulin and a longer-acting insulin to get the blood sugar control you want.

"Regular insulin looks clear and acts in the first few hours after a shot. NPH and Lente insulins look cloudy. They begin to work more slowly but their effect lasts much longer.

"I'll always write your insulin doses so that the units of Regular insulin come first. I want you to think of your doses that way too—first the units of Regular and then the units of NPH. That will remind you to always draw-up the Regular insulin first when you prepare a shot. Drawing up the Regular insulin first keeps you from accidentally mixing any of the longer-acting NPH insulin into the Regular. If that happened, your clear bottle of Regular insulin would turn cloudy. You'd have to throw it away and buy a new bottle. So remember, first draw up R, then N."

"OK, Doc, I'll remember. You were saying that *when* I take my insulin is important. I guess I've never paid much attention to that. I figured as long as I took it pretty close to meal time—either before or after—it was fine."

"But it's not, Mike. Timing is important. Injecting insulin is like shooting skeet. You have to 'lead' the target. That is, you have to shoot ahead of a moving clay pigeon in order to hit it. With insulin, you need to shoot (inject) ahead of the meal—for most people 45 to 60 minutes before the meal. That's the only way to get insulin and food into the bloodstream at the same time."

"But I'll have a reaction if I inject that long before a meal. I've even taken my insulin *after* meals a few times to avoid low blood sugar reactions," Mike said.

"Strange as it sounds," the doctor replied, "NOT leading the meal with your insulin can actually increase your chances for having a low blood sugar reaction."

The young man found that very hard to believe and said so.

"Let me show you what I mean." The doctor drew two graphs on a small piece of paper. Each graph had two curves on it to represent the effects of insulin and food. The doctor pointed to the first graph and continued.

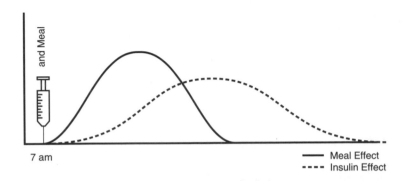

"Not leading the meal with insulin is one way to produce 'curve mismatch.' That's what happens when the major action of your insulin occurs at a different time than the major effect of food from your meal. Having a lot of insulin around when just a little food is available increases your risk for having a low blood sugar reaction.

"Now look at what happens when you lead the target:

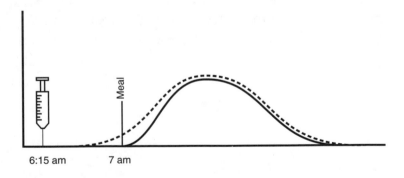

"Notice how the curves match more closely. This produces better blood sugar control."

"You may be right," the young man conceded. "But it still seems that if I waited that long to eat, I'd probably have a reaction. It's happened to me before."

The doctor then explained that it takes quite a while for insulin injected under the skin to be absorbed and to enter the bloodstream. Even more time passes before the blood sugar level actually begins to fall.

"In short, Mike, when you had a reaction right after taking a shot, it was almost certainly caused by the tail end of whatever insulin you had taken PREVIOUSLY, not by the most recent shot."

"Would it make a difference whether I was taking beef, pork, or human insulin?"

"No, it wouldn't make any difference in what you should do. All of this applies regardless of the source of the insulin you're taking. But it might make a difference in how successful we are in controlling your blood sugar."

"Why would it make a difference in my blood sugar? I thought insulin was insulin."

"Insulin *is* insulin, but human bodies are made to use human, not beef or pork, insulin. Your body recognizes insulin from animals as being different from human insulin. And even though the differences are very small, they can cause the body to make chemicals called antibodies that attack the animal insulin. In effect, the antibodies 'tie up' some of the beef or pork insulin so it's not available to lower the blood sugar. This effect can be strong enough in some people to result in poor blood sugar control. So, since one of your goals is better control, today we're going to get you started on Dynamic Insulin Dosing using human insulin. I think you're going to see an improvement in your blood sugars because of these changes."

"OK, Doc, if you say so, I'll give it a try." And off he went, determined to ride this bike called diabetes.

Dynamic Insulin Dosing Guidelines

Dynamic Insulin Dosing is a method for improving blood sugar control by making small changes in insulin doses based on finger-stick blood sugar tests. It is used when there is no illness present to alter insulin requirements and it is based on the following information:

Insulin type	Injected	Has its major effect	Effect is shown by blood sugar test taken
Regular	Before breakfast	Between breakfast and lunch	Before lunch
NPH or Lente	Before breakfast	Between lunch and supper	Before supper
Regular	Before supper	Between supper and bedtime	Before night snack
NPH or Lente	Before supper or at bedtime	Overnight	Before breakfast

Dynamic Insulin Dosing

The following chart of insulin dose changes is based on a blood sugar "action point" of 180. The "action point" is the highest acceptable blood sugar value in each person's desired range of control. If your highest acceptable blood sugar is higher or lower than 180, substitute your own value for 180 in the charts below.

For high blood sugars not caused by illness or extra food intake . . .

If blood sugar is over 180 for three days in a row

Before breakfast:
> THEN, beginning on day 4
> • INCREASE evening NPH* insulin 1 unit.

Before lunch:
> THEN, beginning on day 4
> • INCREASE morning Regular insulin 1 unit.

Before supper:
> THEN, beginning on day 4
> • INCREASE morning NPH* insulin 2 units.

Before bedtime:
> THEN, beginning on day 4
> • INCREASE evening Regular insulin 1 unit.

* or Lente insulin

For low blood sugars not caused by skipped or delayed meals or an increase in physical activity . . .

If the blood sugar is less than 70 or low blood sugar symptoms are present

> *Between bedtime and breakfast:*
> - REDUCE tonight's NPH* insulin 2 units.

> *Between breakfast and lunch:*
> - REDUCE tomorrow morning's Regular insulin 2 units.

> *Between lunch and supper:*
> - REDUCE tomorrow morning's NPH* insulin 3 units.

> *Between supper and bedtime:*
> - REDUCE tomorrow evening's Regular insulin 2 units.

* or Lente insulin

Insulin . . .

—Is needed every day. Missing a single dose
could result in serious problems.

—Is best taken at the same time each day.

—Works best when taken 45 to 60 minutes before
a meal.

—With Dynamic Insulin Dosing and a doctor's
assistance, can produce good blood sugar
control.

4

Feeding the Flames: Nutrition

He likes bread and butter, She likes toast and jam.
—Devo

A few days later the young man returned to the office for his first visit with the diabetes educator.

"I've never heard of a diabetes educator. What do you do exactly?"

"Well, the title is pretty descriptive," she replied. "It's my job to help you learn what you need to know to take control of your diabetes. Most educators are nurses or dietitians specially trained in both diabetes and teaching. We usually work in the offices of doctors who specialize in diabetes or for hospitals that have diabetes education programs."

She continued, "There's a lot to learn about diabetes, and learning takes time—more time than most doctors can really give. So educators are usually the ones to teach people with diabetes about their insulin, what to eat, how to care for their feet, and so on. We'll get to all of those things eventually, but we'll take it one step at a time. Do you know where you'd like to start?"

"Eating!" Mike said. "Trying to figure out what to eat drives me crazy. Lately I've just been avoiding sugar and eating pretty much everything else. But I have a hunch that's not enough. Some foods seem to have a bigger effect than others—even some foods that don't have any sugar in them. But isn't there a simpler way than weighing and measuring everything I eat? I really don't think I can manage that."

"Well, you're right, what you eat IS important in controlling your diabetes," the educator said, "and there's a lot to learn. But let's start with something pretty simple: the basics of WHAT you eat, HOW MUCH you eat, and WHEN you eat it. Later you may want to learn how to read nutrition labels. You may also want to know what kinds of foods can help cut your risk for heart disease or how to read a restaurant menu. Eventually, you'll probably want to learn a meal planning system like carbohydrate counting or exchanges to help you get even better blood sugar control. But for now, we'll start with the basics.

"WHAT to eat is pretty straightforward," she continued. "You don't really need special food products or way-out menus. The same foods that were enjoyable and 'good for you' before you had diabetes are still your best choices. All of us feel our best when we eat regular meals that include vegetables, fruits, grains, and low-fat protein and dairy foods.

"In fact, rather than calling it a Diabetic Diet, let's just call it a Healthy Meal Plan. It's the kind of meal plan that everyone should be on and it includes a lot of options. That's why I don't like to call it a diet. The word 'diet' sounds so rigid. It makes people think that in order to be on it they have to walk around hungry all day. That's not the case at all."

"Well, that's good to hear," Mike said. "Once I had a doctor who gave me a sheet of paper with a low-calorie diabetic diet on it. I went to him because my diabetes was out of control and I was losing weight. But on his diet I lost even more weight and I felt awful. I was hungry all the time. He gave me a low-calorie diet even though I'd never been fat in my life."

"That's what sometimes happens when you get a pre-printed diet sheet. They almost never fit your needs very well. It's important to spend time with a dietitian or a diabetes educator. If you're going to be on a calorie-controlled meal plan, someone who knows what they're doing should choose the calorie level carefully.

"Also, people like different foods. Everyone's taste isn't the same. You can't give all of them the same diet and expect them to do well."

Mike replied, "Well, it sure didn't work for me. Eating right definitely involves a lot more than just avoiding sweets."

"It's part of the picture, Mike. But as you've noticed, avoiding sweets by itself won't give you the control you want. To do that, you need to balance your whole diet with the right insulin plan. Eating large amounts of sugar and fat can contribute to poor blood sugar control and other health problems," the educator explained. "But fat-and sugar-filled foods weren't very good choices BEFORE you had diabetes either.

"Controlling how much sugar and fat you get from food isn't always easy because sometimes the presence of fat and sugar isn't obvious," she pointed out. "But for now, avoid or limit foods that are *obvious* sources of fat and sugar—fried food, gravy, butter, salad dressing, candy, pie, cake frosting, regular soda pop, and so on. When you're ready, learning to read food labels can help you avoid *hidden* fats and sugars as well. Staying away from high-fat and high-sugar foods is a great first step toward a healthier diet.

"The next step is to eat a variety of foods at each meal and snack," the educator continued. "Combinations that provide carbohydrate with small amounts of protein and fat will produce more stable blood sugars."

She handed Mike a piece of paper that read:

**Include foods from both groups
in meals and snacks**

Larger portions of carbohydrate foods	*Smaller portions of low-fat protein foods*
- Bread	- Meat, lean
- Cereal	- Milk,* low-fat
- Potatoes	or skim
- Rice	- Fish
- Beans*	- Chicken
- Crackers	- Low-fat cheese
- Noodles	- Beans*
- Fruit	- Tofu
	- Natural peanut
	butter

For best health, portions of carbohydrate foods should be larger than portions of protein foods. Try to keep carbohydrate portions about the same size from day to day.

*Milk and beans contain both carbohydrate and protein

"I understand," said Mike, "but how much of these foods should I eat?"

"There are two things involved in answering your question," she said.

"The first is the total amount of food you need and the second is the amount you eat at any one time.

"First, let's talk about the total amount of food you need each day. The amount of energy—calories—you need depends on a number of things including your size, your level of physical activity, and whether you're a man or a woman. It ISN'T affected by the fact that you have diabetes or how much insulin you're taking. Simply put, you need enough food every day to keep your body at your best weight. In Type I diabetes—the kind you have—you can't get good blood sugar control by eating less than your body really needs."

This was news to Mike. He'd often tried to eat less when his blood sugars were high. Sometimes he would even skip a snack because of high sugars. It seemed so logical, even though he had to admit it hadn't worked very well.

"You mean some people have a different kind of diabetes than mine? Is that why eating less doesn't work?"

"Yes, on both counts, Mike," the educator replied. "But I think it helps to think of diabetes as something you DON'T have, rather than something you DO. What you DON'T have anymore is the ability to regulate your blood sugar level automatically. What your body used to do for itself now needs to be done from the outside, no matter what kind of diabetes you have."

"How many kinds of diabetes are there?" he asked.

"Several," the educator answered, "But Type I and Type II are the most common. In the past, Type I was called *juvenile diabetes* and Type II diabetes was referred to as *adult-onset.*"

"What's the difference?"

"In Type I diabetes, the cells of the pancreas that make insulin—the beta cells—have been destroyed. We think that their destruction is caused by a problem with the immune system. The immune system's job is to protect us from invading germs. In some people, the system seems to get 'confused' and attacks cells that make insulin as if they were invaders. We don't know why this happens, but the result is that these people lose the ability to make insulin. Because of this they have to take insulin shots every day.

"Type II diabetes is a different disease," she continued. "Many people with this kind of diabetes make as much insulin as people who don't have diabetes. Sometimes they even make more! The problem is that their insulin isn't used effectively.

"Remember how the doctor explained that insulin keeps the door to the log cabin open so that fuel can be brought in to feed the fire? You can think of a cabin belonging to someone with Type II diabetes as having rusty hinges, making the door hard to open. This type of diabetes can often be treated with a healthy meal plan, exercise, and pills. All of these treatments help in some way to 'oil' the rusty hinges so the door works better and insulin can do its job."

"Those pills sound a lot better than taking shots," Mike said. "Can I switch to those if I'm really careful about my food and exercise?"

"A good thought, Mike, but I'm afraid it won't work. The diabetes pills aren't insulin. They just help insulin that's already in the body to work better."

"But why can't they make pills that have insulin in them?"

"If you took insulin by mouth, it would be digested like food and lose its ability to lower blood sugar."

"How about people with Type II diabetes?" he wanted to know. "Do they ever have to take shots?"

"Some do and some don't," the educator answered. "The first thing that we try is a healthy low-calorie meal plan and an increase in exercise. If that doesn't bring the blood sugar down to normal, we add one of those diabetes pills. If the blood sugars are still above normal with a good program of diet, exercise, and pills, we usually add insulin to the treatment plan. Now that you understand some of the differences between Type I and Type II diabetes, are you ready to get back to your original question about food?"

"Yes, I am." Mike settled back in his chair.

The educator reminded him, "When we got sidetracked, we had been talking about how much food you need each day. Remember that with Type I diabetes you need as much food every day as it takes to maintain a healthy weight; starving yourself isn't a good way to get your blood sugars under control. Blood sugar control comes from matching your insulin to the amount of food you actually need every day.

"Now let's talk about how much you should eat at one time," the educator continued. "Think again about building a fire in the fireplace of your cabin. If you were depending on that fire to keep you warm all through a freezing winter's night, you wouldn't throw all of the wood on the fire at once."

"Why not?" he asked.

"Because, if you did that, the fire would blaze madly for awhile, and quickly burn up all of the logs. The fire would probably be out before morning. But if you took the same amount of wood and fed it to the fire slowly throughout the night, in the morning you'd still have a nice warm fire. You might even have some logs left over."

She explained further, "Eating to help control your diabetes is like feeding logs to that fire a few at a time. Dividing up your food among several meals and snacks will keep the fire burning evenly. You'll have a warm, well controlled fire all through the day and night, instead of a raging inferno that later goes out because of a lack of fuel.

"Now with your insulin program of two shots containing both Regular and NPH insulin, you actually have four times when the insulin peaks."

She drew a small picture to show Mike when his insulins act.

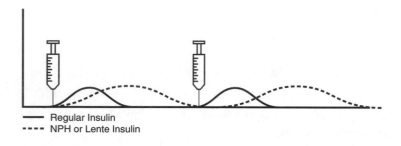

——— Regular Insulin
- - - - NPH or Lente Insulin

"Your insulin peaks for breakfast, lunch and dinner, but, as you can see, there's also a fair amount of insulin around between meals. So for you, eating breakfast, lunch, and dinner, with snacks at mid-morning, mid-afternoon, and bedtime is most likely to keep your blood sugar stable: no big blazes and no times when the fire sputters out for lack of fuel. Different patterns of meals and snacks work better with different insulin regimens. So if either your meal pattern or your insulin plan change, the other has to change as well."

"But isn't that a lot of food?" Mike wanted to know. "Seems like I'll gain weight on three meals AND three snacks."

The educator smiled. "Don't worry, Mike. I'm not suggesting that you have to eat more. I'm just recommending that we change the way you divide up the amount of food you normally eat. You'll still be eating the same total amount of food. But by dividing it up into three meals and three snacks, you'll get better blood sugar control and protect yourself against low blood sugar reactions. First, I'd like you to tell me about the usual size of your meals. Then we'll create the snacks by borrowing food from the meals."

"OK, so you're not trying to ruin my figure," he said. "And I'll actually be glad to try the snacks if they'll cut down on these miserable low blood sugars. Saying that reminds me of something I don't understand. Why is my blood sugar lower on an afternoon when I have a steak and salad for lunch instead of my usual sandwich and milk? I know the steak has more calories."

The educator complimented Mike on being so observant and then explained, "The starches and sugars in high carbohydrate foods, like the bread and milk in your usual lunch, are all converted to blood sugar—100 percent. The steak doesn't contain any carbohydrate, only protein and fat. About half of the calories from the protein and less than 15 percent of the fat end up as blood sugar. So even though the steak has more calories, it has less impact on the blood sugar level. And after you eat the steak you have a reaction because the insulin dose you took in the morning matches the amount of carbohydrate in your usual lunch. The steak isn't your usual lunch.

"To keep your meals and insulin in balance," she went on," you need to eat similar servings of bread, cereal, pasta, milk, fruit, and other carbohydrate foods at about the same time each day. Having twice as much fruit at breakfast or half as much bread at lunch will make a big difference in your blood sugar. That's because the change in carbohydrate intake destroys the balance between your food and insulin."

"So what I eat really does make a difference. Does it matter *when* I eat, too? Mike asked.

"Yes, it really does. That old saying 'Timing is everything' is certainly true of diabetes," the educator answered.

Mike mentioned the doctor's advice that he eat 45 to 60 minutes after taking his insulin. "I should have my merit badge in skeet shooting by now," he said. "I'm a master at leading the target."

"Well, that's a great start," the educator replied, "but it's not the only concern. Waiting *too long* to eat can cause just as many problems as not waiting long enough."

"Oh, I know that," Mike said. "If I don't get lunch by 12:15, I'm sure to have a reaction. I'm careful to eat on time, especially when my blood sugars are on the low side."

"What would you say if I told you it's just as important to be careful about timing when your blood sugar's on the high side?" she asked.

"I'd say I'm about through being surprised at anything you tell me," Mike replied.

The educator then described what can happen when people delay eating because their blood sugar is high before a meal. She explained that some people keep testing their blood sugar until their insulin brings the blood sugar down. They won't start eating until the blood sugar is in the normal range.

"This amounts to throwing a big log on the fire at the wrong time," she said. "It can cause a big upward swing in blood sugars later in the day because of 'curve mismatch.' The delayed meal creates a big demand for insulin AFTER the insulin's strongest action is past."

"I eat less when my blood sugar is high," said Mike. "Like last night. My blood sugar was 236 at bedtime, so I skipped my bedtime snack. I don't think it's a good idea to push a high blood sugar even higher by eating."

"I know that sounds logical, Mike. But remember the story about feeding logs to the fire gradually to keep it going all night. When you skip your bedtime snack, you increase your chances for having a reaction in the middle of the night."

Mike wrinkled his forehead. "Do you mean having a high blood sugar at bedtime doesn't protect me from having a reaction overnight?"

"Don't count on it. Remember that your overall goal is to match food peaks and insulin peaks. A blood sugar peak at bedtime doesn't match up with the peak of your insulin that acts overnight. That peak comes hours later. After all, 12 to 15 hours can go by between your evening meal and breakfast. The night snack is really important—even when your sugar is higher than you want it to be at bedtime."

Mike was shaking his head. "Gee, when I came in here today I thought the most important thing about my diet was avoiding sweets. It's definitely more complicated than that. Not only do I have to think about choosing the food, but I also have to pay attention to how much I eat and when I eat it."

"Definitely," she said. "But the more you learn, the more foods you'll be able to enjoy without disturbing your diabetes control. For now, concentrate on choosing a healthy variety of foods and eating about the same amount at the same time each day. We'll write down some menus based on your usual meals to help you with that. Later on, when the rest of your basic education about diabetes is done, we'll move on to more advanced approaches."

Nutrition Basics

1. Good diabetes control starts with a varied and healthful meal plan.

2. Eat enough food to maintain your best weight. If you're losing weight without dieting, check your diabetes control.

3. Eat about the same amount of food at the same time each day. Delaying or skipping meals and changing the amount of food eaten can destroy the balance between food and insulin.

4. Keep learning about food and diabetes. The more you know, the more choices you have.

5. A personalized meal plan prepared just for you by a registered dietitian who specializes in diabetes can make living successfully with diabetes much more enjoyable.

5

Installing the Altimeter: Monitoring

We can float among the stars together, you and I,
And we can fly.
— The Fifth Dimension

After Mike had mastered the basics of insulin and food, he and the educator concentrated on how to monitor his diabetes. She told him they would be checking three different measures of diabetes control. Two of them would be his responsibility.

"Let's start with blood sugar tests. I know you've been doing finger-stick blood sugars for quite a while, Mike. Now let's talk about how you can use them to really make a difference in your blood sugar control."

"I'll bet you've got another story," the young man observed.

"How'd you guess?" she replied. "Controlling your diabetes is not only like riding a bike. In some ways it's also like flying an airplane. A pilot flying at 5,000 feet checks his altimeter to find out whether he's the right distance from the ground. And he doesn't just check it once. He checks it repeatedly, because a single reading could be misleading."

"What do you mean?"

"If he glanced at his altimeter only once and it read 5,000 feet, he could assume he's flying straight and level at the desired altitude. But that single reading could also mean he was passing through 5,000 feet on his way up into the stratosphere. Worse yet, he could be diving through 5,000 feet, toward a close encounter of the painful kind with the ground.

"A good pilot takes a series of altimeter readings to make sure that he's flying straight and level. Blood sugar readings work the same way. A single reading—whether it's low, normal, or high—doesn't tell you all that you need to know. To find out whether you're flying straight and level within your desired range of blood sugars, you have to take readings in sequence. Then you can see patterns."

"So, what would you like me to do?"

"I recommend that you test four times each day—before meals and at bedtime."

"That's a lot!" Mike replied.

"I know, but it's the way to find out what your blood sugar is doing all through the day."

"I got really burned out on blood testing. Lately I've only been testing in the morning and when I feel high or low."

"I won't pretend that what I'm asking is easy, Mike. But you'll get a much better picture of your overall control by testing four times in one day than you would by testing four times on four different days. The reason for this is that your blood sugar level changes during the day. Just because you have a normal reading in the morning doesn't mean that your readings will be normal during the rest of the day, too. You've told me you want to keep your blood sugars near normal so you can feel your best and reduce your risk of complications. If that's still your goal, try to keep the readings between 80 and 180 most of the time. Once your level of control stabilizes in that range, we'll know we've worked out the correct match among your insulin, food, and exercise."

"It'll be great to have my diabetes in control once and for all," said Mike.

The educator shook her head. "I have to be honest with you, Mike. That's not going to happen. Getting your diabetes under control is more like a journey than a destination. You're always on the road. Your life and your diabetes are a little different every day. That means that blood testing, watching your food and Dynamic Dosing have to go on all the time to keep your blood sugar near normal."

"It never lets up, does it?"

"No, it doesn't. But even if *diabetes* never lets up, *you* may need to lighten up occasionally! Testing four times a day is what's needed to keep your blood sugars in really good control. It's what the doctor and I recommend: the ideal. But I'll also tell you that I've never had a patient who stuck to that ideal 100 percent of the time. If you feel like the demands of taking care of your diabetes are really weighing you down, it may be better to relax and lighten up a bit: test less frequently for a while or have a piece of cake on your birthday. It doesn't have to be the biggest piece of cake. When you do those things, your blood sugar control will probably slip. But that may be an acceptable price to pay in the short term to protect your motivation to keep at it over the long haul.

"If you do cut back on testing occasionally, I suggest that you still test four times a day at least one day a week. This will help make sure things don't get too badly out of control while you're taking your break. Remember, four tests in one day always tell us more about your control than four tests done on four different days."

"So less testing means less control," Mike observed, "but testing four times a day will keep my blood sugars in line."

"It's a big help," she agreed, "but don't expect your blood sugars to ALWAYS be in the target range, even when you've done everything 'by the book.' Occasional unexplained high blood sugars are just part of having diabetes. The goal isn't to get perfect blood sugar readings. That's just not possible. Instead, the goal is to get the majority of your blood sugar readings in the target range most of the time. That's why we use blood sugar PATTERNS to adjust your insulin, instead of responding to a single high reading.

"Also, Mike, remember that there's no such thing as a 'bad' blood sugar. Your blood sugar record only contains pieces of information. Whether a reading is above, below, or within your target range, it's still useful information you can act on to maintain or improve your diabetes control."

Mike hesitated, then said, "That sounds good in theory, but I think I'll still feel disappointed when my blood sugars are way off the mark."

"That's only natural. But disappointment is different than guilt. Feeling like there's something wrong with *you* just because your blood sugar is out of range doesn't help matters. I'd much rather see you focus on doing something with the numbers than on beating yourself up about the fact that they're there.

"Now let's talk about the second sort of test that we'd like you to do regularly: urine testing."

"Urine tests?" asked the young man. "I thought those were obsolete now that we do finger-stick blood sugars. I know for a fact that urine sugar tests aren't very accurate."

"You're absolutely right. Urine tests for sugar really AREN'T very accurate as a way of knowing what your blood sugar is," the educator agreed. "But we recommend you test your urine, not just for sugar, but also for ketones." (See "Interpreting Morning Urine Tests for Sugar and Ketones" on page 53 for help understanding the results of this test.)

"What's a ketone?"

"Ketones are chemicals that show up in the urine when your diabetes is getting out of control. Blood sugar testing doesn't tell you whether you're producing ketones or not because blood glucose meters can't measure them.

"That's why we recommend urine ketone testing for everyone who has Type I diabetes. We also suggest that people with Type II diabetes who take insulin do this test when they're sick. Later I'll give you guidelines for how to use urine ketone test results. For now, all I want you to realize is that urine testing for sugar and ketones is part of our overall plan for keeping track of your diabetes."

"OK, I can wait. But you said there was a third kind of test I should know about."

"It's called a glycosylated hemoglobin test. Years ago, the only tool a doctor had to judge how well someone's diabetes was being controlled was a fasting blood sugar. The doctor did one of these every few weeks or months. They had serious drawbacks."

"Really?"

"Yes. Their main weakness was how little information they gave the doctor. It was almost impossible to recommend helpful changes in the insulin dose or diet based on a single fasting blood sugar reading. And just as important, they couldn't give the doctor a clear picture of how well the management plan was working. There wasn't any way to know what the 'average' blood sugar had been since the last visit.

"And, for the person with diabetes, going into the doctor's office to have blood drawn for a fasting blood sugar was far from ideal. The best that he or she could expect was a hungry morning spent waiting for the blood draw. Sometimes the doctor was delayed, making it even harder. Most of the time, the patient's routine was badly upset because he waited to take his insulin until after he'd seen the doctor. Of course, that would throw off the timing of meals and insulin for the whole day. The blood sugars would almost certainly go out of control. We've talked before about how critical timing is to controlling your diabetes."

"I know," Mike said. "I've been in that situation more than once."

"These days, finger-stick blood sugar tests give us a lot more information. And it's information that's especially helpful in managing day-to-day changes in food, insulin, and activity.

"But each finger-stick blood sugar, just like a fasting blood sugar, only measures one point in time. Before you developed diabetes, your pancreas was constantly measuring your blood sugar and adding the right amounts of insulin to your bloodstream 24 hours per day. I know that doing four finger-sticks a day seems like a lot. But it still only tells us what's happening at four split seconds during the day.

"You know how much blood sugars can vary. Because of this, even though they're so helpful, your blood tests still may not reveal a true picture of your overall blood sugar control."

"So what do we do?"

"Well, that's where the glycosylated hemoglobin test comes in. It allows us to see what the blood sugar control has been like over the past several weeks."

"I know hemoglobin has something to do with the blood," Mike said, "but what in the world is *glycosylated*?"

"Picture one of your red blood cells as an apple," the educator answered. "If we dipped the apple in sugar syrup, it would come out coated with a certain amount of sugar.

The thicker the syrup, the thicker the coating of sugar on our candied apple.

"Red blood cells have a life span of about 120 days. As they move around the body in the bloodstream, they pick up more or less 'sugar coating,' depending on the amount of sugar in the blood. That sugar-coating process is called glycosylation. It's going on every minute of every day.

"By taking a blood sample every so often and sending it to the lab, we can, in a sense, check the amount of sugar coating on the candied apple. If there was a lot of sugar in the bloodstream during the last few weeks, the glycosylated hemoglobin will be above normal. If the average blood sugar level was in the target range, the glycosylated hemoglobin will be lower. Our goal is a reading as close to the normal range as possible."

"You mean the same reading as for a person who doesn't have diabetes?"

"Yes, or close to it."

Mike left the office thinking what a change it was to be working with people who listened. He enjoyed having his questions answered in ways he could understand.

Monitoring

1. Finger-stick blood sugars before meals and at bedtime show your pattern of blood sugar control.

2. Patterns tell you far more than any single blood sugar value.

3. Testing urine for sugar and ketones can provide additional helpful information.

4. Glycosylated hemoglobin helps reveal overall diabetes control.

Interpreting Morning Urine Tests for Sugar and Ketones

The following chart explains the results of urine tests for sugar and ketones. It is based on testing the *first* urine passed in the morning. The guidelines are true for people who begin to show sugar in the urine when their blood sugar gets higher than 180. This is true for most people, but exceptions do occur.

- *Negative Sugar/Negative Ketones*
Overnight blood sugar stayed between about 70 and 180. This is the goal.

- *Negative Sugar/Positive Ketones*
Overnight blood sugar did not go over 180. Ketones indicate a low blood sugar reaction may have occurred.

- *Positive Sugar/Negative Ketones*
Overnight blood sugar went above 180.

- *Positive Sugar/Positive Ketones*
Overnight blood sugar went above 180, and the ketones indicate your diabetes is getting out of control.

6

When the Fire Goes Out: Hypoglycemia

As the miller told his tale, her face—at first just
ghostly—turned a whiter shade of pale.
                                                    Procol Harum

Time passed. Mike's blood sugars were improving. They were lower than they'd ever been since he developed diabetes—so much lower, in fact, that he was having a lot of low blood sugar reactions. He was frustrated. If good control meant having reactions nearly every day, he didn't want any part of it.

"I'm really sick of insulin reactions!" he complained to the doctor. "I feel so rotten when my sugar bottoms out that I'm tempted to keep it on the high side. I never had this many reactions when my blood sugars were high. Now that I'm in tight control, I feel worse than ever."

"But you're not in tight control, Mike," the doctor explained. "Having frequent reactions means your diabetes is out of control—out of control on the low side. When we started working together, your diabetes was out of control on the high side. Your reactions are telling us that we overshot the mark. But there is a solution. You need the next installment in the saga of the log cabin to understand how low blood sugars happen and how to prevent them."

He reminded Mike that insulin holds the cabin door open so wood can be brought in to feed the fire. Then he asked what would happen if the supply of wood ran out.

"Well, the fire would go out," he replied.

"And that's exactly what happens when there isn't enough food around when your insulin is acting. The body's energy-producing fire goes out. The body recognizes this situation as a real threat. It tries to correct the problem by releasing certain chemicals called hormones that raise the blood sugar: glucagon, epinephrine, growth hormone, and others. Besides raising your blood sugar, they can cause some pretty uncomfortable symptoms.

"What kind of symptoms do you have when your blood sugar gets low?" the doctor asked.

"I usually get shaky and break out in a sweat," the young man answered. "But there have been times when I've gotten confused and was kind of bumbling around."

The doctor explained to Mike that it's important for each person to know and watch out for his or her own particular symptoms of a falling blood sugar level.

"Symptoms can range from weakness and shakiness to headaches or tingling around the mouth and lips. In fact, low blood sugar reactions can cause almost any symptom that your body can have. For instance, stomachaches, dizziness, and feeling nervous can all be caused by low blood sugars. That's why it's a good idea to check your sugar anytime you're not feeling right. That's the only way to tell for sure whether or not you're having a reaction."

The doctor continued, "The symptoms can get pretty severe. When you lose your coordination or get confused, it's a sign the brain isn't getting enough fuel. You might even pass out if a reaction that severe goes untreated."

"That's scary," Mike said.

"You're right about that. And the scariest part is how a reaction that severe could lead to a serious accident if it happened while you were driving or climbing a ladder or doing something similar. Besides, repeated severe reactions can cause brain damage. At the very least, reactions make you feel awful. And in the worst case, they put you in real danger."

"What can I do about it?"

"Quite a bit, actually," the doctor replied. "Most reactions can be prevented by just applying what you already know about how food, insulin, and activity affect your blood sugar."

"Remember when we first met, I compared managing your diabetes to riding a two-wheel bike? Well, if you keep everything centered when you're riding the bike, you keep your balance and pedal along without any problems. But if you lean too far one way or the other, the bike falls over.

"It's the same with diabetes. Think of skipping a snack, delaying a meal, or changing the time you take your insulin like leaning too far over on the bike. All of these can produce curve mismatch—a situation where your insulin and food curves don't match—setting you up for a low blood sugar reaction."

"But what should I do if I do have one," the young man asked. "I usually feel terrible when it happens. And it seems to take so long before I begin to feel better. I generally end up stuffing myself before I feel human again."

"In an insulin reaction, the fire is going out. You need to get it going again as quickly as you can. So use something that burns fast and hot. It's like using newspapers or small twigs to start the fire in the cabin's fireplace. High sugar foods that are quickly digested act like 'newspaper.' Glucose gel or tablets, fruit juice, and regular soda pop are best because they act quickest. Some of my patients even carry small tubes of cake icing. Hard candy and fruit will also do the job.

"Quick-acting sugars will help you feel better faster than other foods, but they only support the blood sugar for a short time—sort of like newspapers that help start the fire but won't keep it going for very long. So, if the next meal is more than an hour away, you'll need to put a 'log' on the fire."

"What's a log?" Mike asked.

"Logs are foods like peanut butter sandwiches, meat sandwiches, or cheese and crackers. They contain carbohydrate, protein, and fat. They release sugar into the bloodstream more slowly than fruit juice and other high-sugar foods. This helps prevent you from having another insulin reaction before the next meal rolls around."

"I usually just move up the time of my next meal. That gives me logs, right?"

"It gives you logs all right," the doctor agreed, "but it's not the best way to handle a reaction. Changing the time of your meal increases your risk of having another reaction later on."

"What do you mean?"

"Let's say you usually eat supper at 6 p.m. But today at 4:30, you have an insulin reaction. So you decide to eat supper then because you're feeling low."

"I've done that."

"So far so good, but the problem comes a little later in the evening. On a normal day, the food from your 6 p.m. supper would match up with the insulin you inject at about 5:15. But today you ate your supper at 4:30 because of the reaction. By the time your evening insulin begins to peak, your supper is digested and long gone. You're probably going to run out of fuel and have another reaction later that evening."

"I've done that, too! So, I'll do better if I eat my meals at the usual times, but treat reactions with 'newspaper and logs?'"

"Right," the doctor agreed. "By the way, keep in mind you won't always feel symptoms when your blood sugar is getting too low."

"I learned that the hard way," Mike said. "Last spring I had a reaction that came on without warning. I literally didn't know what hit me until I woke up to find myself looking into the eyes of a big, sweaty paramedic."

"I'll bet that was excitement you could have done without," the doctor said. "That's called an *asymptomatic* reaction, meaning you didn't have any symptoms. It happens if your body doesn't release those hormones we talked about when your blood sugar starts to fall. Asymptomatic reactions are more common in people whose blood sugars have been in poor control for many years. But you know from your own experience, they can happen to other people, too.

"Because you can't always rely on getting symptoms when your blood sugar is too low, my advice is to treat any blood sugar of 70 or less with 'newspapers and logs.'"

"Why do you pick 70?"

"Because home blood glucose meters are only accurate to within 10 to 15 percent of the actual blood sugar value. They'll get you 'in the ball park' but won't necessarily give you the exact value. For example, if we sent your blood sample to the lab and got back the exact blood sugar value of 100, your meter could show any value between 85 and 115 and still be working just fine."

"But, Doc, that's quite a spread."

"That's the best you can do with these machines."

"You've got to be kidding. That doesn't sound very good."

"It's good enough to keep you in control of your blood sugar. There is another choice, though. If you like, you could spend $35,000 on the kind of machine the lab uses and carry it around with you in a moving van."

"Very cute, but I think I'll stick with my meter."

"Wise choice. Meters are great, Mike, but they're not perfect," the doctor went on. "We just need to use what we know about how precise they are. For example, in the case of a finger-stick blood sugar reading of 70, the true blood sugar could actually be lower, as low as the high 50's. So rather than risk a crash, I recommend you treat any blood sugar of 70 or lower immediately—even if you feel just fine."

"Immediately?" Mike asked. "Even if I'm doing something important, like trying to make it to a business appointment on time?"

"Yes. Begin treatment immediately, at the first sign of a reaction. The longer you wait, the worse the reaction can get and the harder it can be to treat. Also keep in mind that sometimes it's possible to have a low blood sugar reaction with a blood sugar above 70. So if you're having symptoms of a low blood sugar reaction but your blood test comes out between 70 and 100, go ahead and treat it with 'newspaper.' If you feel better after treating it, then you know that was the reason why you were feeling bad. If there isn't a change in how you feel, that wasn't the problem."

"So, Doc, let me see if I have this straight. If my blood sugar is below 70, I should treat it immediately no matter whether I feel symptoms or not. When my blood sugar is between 70 and 100, I should only treat it if I have symptoms; but if I'm feeling good, I should leave it alone."

"That's right, Mike. And, please, begin treatment right away, even if it means getting to an appointment late. I think it's better to arrive a little late than to get somewhere confused or not at all because of a bad reaction."

"You mean like the one I had when I passed out. Could I have done anything to save that visit from the paramedic?"

"Yes, that was definitely a severe reaction. In a case like that, glucagon could have helped."

"Glucagon?" Mike asked. "What's that?"

"It's a hormone that works opposite to insulin. A shot of insulin moves sugar out of the bloodstream and into the cells, causing the blood sugar to fall. A shot of glucagon moves sugar out of the liver and into the bloodstream, causing the blood sugar level to rise. Glucagon is the best treatment for a severe low blood sugar reaction that makes you pass out or has you so confused you can't even swallow.

"Even though your blood sugar will go up after a glucagon shot, don't expect it to happen right away. After it's injected, it may be 10 to 15 minutes before the blood sugar starts to rise and you wake up. Once you're awake, the glucagon should be followed up with 'newspaper and logs.'"

The doctor gave Mike a prescription for a Glucagon Emergency Kit. "Get a couple now, before you need them. Keep your glucagon in an easy-to-find place at home and at work. Your friends, family, and close co-workers should learn how to use it. They're the ones you'll be relying on to use it if you should ever have another severe reaction. It needs to be mixed just before it's used. It's injected just like insulin."

"Doc, is there anytime that I would inject glucagon myself, rather than having someone else do it?"

"Yes, there is, Mike. If you ever get sick to your stomach and are throwing up a lot, glucagon could come in very handy.

"If you had a low blood sugar reaction under those circumstances, it would be hard to treat it with food. You probably couldn't keep anything down. In that case, you could give yourself a shot of glucagon to pull yourself out of the reaction. But if that ever happens, give me a call. If you're throwing up and having reactions, we need to be sure that we can keep your blood sugar up."

"How would you do that?"

"I'd hook you up to a bottle of sugar water and have it run into a vein in your arm. That would stop your blood sugar from going any lower."

"Why couldn't I just keep using glucagon?"

"Because glucagon can't be used very often. You see, Mike, the liver is like a warehouse full of sugar. Glucagon opens the doors of the warehouse and lets the sugar out. Once that sugar is gone, there isn't any left to replace it. If you went into another reaction fairly soon, giving another shot of glucagon might not help because the warehouse would be empty. We need to refill it—replace the stored sugar that the glucagon released. Once you stop throwing up, you can refill it by eating. But while you're still throwing up, we have to refill it by giving you sugar through a vein in your arm."

"I guess the bottom line is to take my meals and insulin on time to prevent reactions but prepare for any reactions that might still come along."

"That's right, Mike."

"But, Doc, how could I have planned in advance for this problem? Once I took my morning dose of insulin at night by mistake, rather than my nighttime dose, which was much smaller."

"Mike, that happens more often than you might think. Because you can't get the insulin out of you once it's in there, you need to eat some extra food to balance it. If that ever happens again, check your blood sugar and eat a snack every three hours during the night."

"In other words, I need to eat my way through it."

"That's right. And, Mike, one last reminder. Don't forget to wear your diabetes identification at all times. It could save your life if you're ever found unconscious. While it's best to keep the bike balanced, it's still a smart idea to wear a helmet, just in case."

Treat Low Blood Sugars with "Newspaper and Logs"

1. IDENTIFY THE REACTION
- Be aware that any symptom might be caused by a low blood sugar.
- Know your own usual symptoms of a low blood sugar reaction.
- Do a finger-stick blood sugar if you're not sure.

2. BEGIN TREATMENT IMMEDIATELY
- If your blood sugar is 70 or less, begin treatment immediately whether you're having symptoms or not.
- If your blood sugar is between 70 and 100, treat only if you're having symptoms.
- Delay allows the reaction to become more severe and harder to treat.
- Delay can result in unconsciousness.

3. START THE FIRE WITH "NEWSPAPER"
- Eat two or three glucose tablets or one package of glucose gel.
    OR
- Drink eight ounces (or more) of fruit juice or regular soda pop.
- If none of the above is available, eat anything sweet.
- Eat the next meal on time. Don't eat it early because of the reaction.

4. KEEP THE FIRE GOING WITH "LOGS"
- If the next meal or snack is less than an hour away, no "logs" are needed.
- If the next meal or snack is more than an hour away, TREAT AS ABOVE, then add a "log" to the fire.
- Logs are foods that provide carbohydrate, protein, and fat, such as:
    —a meat, cheese or peanut butter sandwich
    —a glass of milk.

5. PREPARE IN ADVANCE FOR SEVERE REACTIONS RESULTING IN LOSS OF CONSCIOUSNESS
- Obtain a GLUCAGON EMERGENCY KIT.
- Instruct family and friends in its use.
- If you pass out, they should inject glucagon immediately.

6. ALWAYS WEAR YOUR DIABETES IDENTIFICATION

7

Burning the Furniture: Sick Days

I got the rockin' pneumonia and
the boogie woogie flu.
Huey "Piano" Smith and the Clowns

The next few weeks passed peacefully. Mike was finally beginning to feel he had control over his diabetes, instead of the other way around. He had a few low blood sugar reactions, but they were mild and he was prepared to treat them. He was absorbed in his daily activities at home and at work. And his blood sugars were right where he wanted them to be. Most were in the target range that he and the doctor had agreed on. Life was going well. He had his old pep back. As he walked into the diabetes educator's office, he almost shouted out the good news.

"This is the best part of my job, Mike. It's great to see what a change you've made using the information we've talked about. I'm delighted you're so satisfied with the results, too.

"But our work's not over," she continued. "Now that you've learned to ride the bike on the straight and narrow, it's time to get ready for obstacles. You need a plan for riding the bike when the weather turns bad—when you get sick."

"But I'm fine," he protested. "Why do I need to think about getting sick now? I just want to enjoy this big improvement."

"I understand that," she replied. "But once you're sick, it's too late to do everything possible to make the situation better. By being prepared, you can keep a garden-variety illness like the flu or a cold from destroying the control you've worked so hard to achieve."

"OK, you win. I'm ready for another story. Am I going to ride the bike, go flying, or return to the log cabin?"

"The log cabin. How about if I go with you this time and keep you company?" she offered. "Let's pretend we're in the log cabin on a freezing winter's night. We're relaxing in front of the fire, talking about something other than diabetes."

"Well, at least we took a break."

"Yes, but the fire is dying down, and we've used up all the firewood you brought in earlier. You head for the door to bring in more wood from outside, but there's been a fierce storm and the door is blocked by ice and snow. It won't budge."

"Things are going from bad to worse here! What else can go wrong?"

"You try the windows, but they're frozen shut, too. The cabin's getting cold.The fireplace flames are sputtering."

"Sounds like a real crisis," Mike said. "What do we do now?"

"We've got to keep warm. We'll freeze if we let the fire go out. So there's only one thing left to do."

"What's that?" Mike asked.

"We'll have to burn the furniture to keep warm. And so we start to pitch it into the fireplace. Obviously, this isn't a perfect solution. The furniture has paint, varnish, and stain on it. It's a different kind of wood than the firewood. It gives off choking black smoke as it's burning. The wood from the woodpile gave off clean white smoke. But at least we'll stay warm until morning."

"Saved by cheap chairs and our own ingenuity!" he said.

"You're really getting into this, Mike. But don't forget there's a point to the story. Think of the storm as an illness—a cold, the flu, or other infection. More strength is needed to hold a door open when a stormy wind is blowing. In the same way, during an illness, the cells of the body have a harder time holding open their cell doors so sugar can enter and be burned for energy.

"Without the fuel provided by sugar, the cell needs to find another way to keep its energy-producing fire going. So it 'burns the furniture.' In this case the furniture is the fat inside the cell. When fat is burned for energy without sugar being available to burn with it, ketones are produced. They're just as noticeable as the black smoke from the burning furniture in the cabin."

"I've been sick a few times since I've had diabetes," said Mike, "but I've never seen any 'black smoke.'"

"That's because you weren't testing for ketones in the past. Now we have you test whenever your blood sugar's over 240 so you'll notice as soon as possible if you're 'burning the furniture.' If that happens, we need to bring it to a halt as soon as we can."

"Why do we need to stop it?" the young man wondered. "Most people probably have plenty of 'furniture' to burn."

"It's important because, just like black smoke from burning the furniture in the cabin polluted the air, large amounts of ketones can be dangerous too. They will eventually make the whole body too acidic. The combination of too much sugar building up in the bloodstream with ketones and excess acid is a life-threatening condition called diabetic ketoacidosis. We call it DKA for short."

"I don't like the sound of 'life threatening,' even if it *does* have a nickname. So what should I do if I find I'm burning the furniture?"

"Here's a list of several things to do when you're sick," the educator answered. "Let's start with your insulin."

"I know I have to take my insulin every day without fail, but shouldn't I reduce the dose when I'm sick and not able to eat as much as usual?" the young man asked.

"No, but that's a common mistake," she answered.

"Remember that when you're sick, the storm is raging, making it harder for the doors to the cells to remain open. That's why you need to take at least your usual amount of insulin. In fact, you may need to take extra insulin on top of your usual dose just to keep those doors open. If the doors don't open, sugar will begin to rise in the bloodstream because it can't get into the cells.

"Also, when you're sick, a number of hormones released by the body can raise the blood sugar level even more."

"But how can that happen if I don't eat?" asked Mike.

"Besides being a warehouse where sugar is stored, the liver is also a factory. It can actually make new sugar under certain conditions. The factory makes and releases sugar at a much higher rate when we're sick than when we're well. It doesn't need food to do that. So even if you haven't eaten a thing, you might find your blood sugar getting higher because of the liver."

"How do you stop the liver from doing that?"

"You use insulin. Insulin will slow down the sugar-producing factory in the liver and help bring things under control," she explained.

"I get it. Not taking your insulin when you're sick can make matters worse by allowing the liver to make all that extra sugar."

"Exactly. That's another reason why it's vital to always take at least your normal dose of insulin and never skip a dose, even when you're sick and can't eat. In fact, the doctor may have you supplement your usual dose with extra Regular insulin when you're sick. (See "Supplements of Regular Insulin for Sick Days, page 76.) When the storm is raging, you may need extra insulin to keep the sugars under control and correct the ketones. But the most important thing to remember is to stay in close contact with the doctor's office whenever you're sick."

When You're Sick

1. Take at least your usual dose of insulin. **Cutting back or skipping a dose of insulin can cause significant problems when you're sick.** Add supplements of Regular insulin as indicated.

2. Use "Foods for Sick Days" (page 77) if you're unable to eat your usual meals.

3. Test a double-voided* urine sample for ketones four times a day at the times of your usual finger-stick blood sugar readings.

4. Report vomiting episodes to your doctor immediately.
   • Take medicine to control vomiting or diarrhea as directed.
   • Drink extra fluids (small frequent sips).
   • Use broth or fruit drinks to replace the fluids and minerals lost during vomiting and diarrhea.

5. Maintain contact with your doctor.

6. Know when your doctor wants you to call.

7. Know how to reach your doctor, especially during non-office hours.

8. If your illness continues or worsens and you can't reach your doctor, go to an emergency room.

*See page 81 for a description of how to obtain a double-voided urine sample.

Supplements of Regular Insulin for Sick Days

When you're sick, your need for insulin may increase. If this happens, your blood sugar level will begin to rise. To correct this problem, **add supplements of Regular insulin to your usual doses** until your blood sugars return to normal. The size of the supplement is based on your blood sugar level. If you have ketones in your urine, *double* the supplement shown for your blood sugar level. Take supplements before meals, but *not* at bedtime. Extra insulin taken at bedtime could cause a reaction while you're asleep and unable to treat it.

Record all supplemental doses in your log book. Begin taking supplements as soon as you recognize that illness has disturbed your diabetes control. Do not take supplements at other times without consulting your doctor.

For a blood sugar of ...	*Add to normal insulin dose:*
Less than 200	0 units of Regular
200 to 249	1 unit of Regular
250 to 299	2 units of Regular
300 to 349	3 units of Regular
350 to 399	4 units of Regular
400 or more	5 units of Regular

Double the supplement if ketones are in the urine

Note: Unless advised differently by your doctor, only use supplemental regular insulin when you're sick. When you're well, make insulin adjustments using the Dynamic Insulin Dosing Guidelines.

Foods for Sick Days

When you're not feeling well enough to eat as you usually do, it's still very important to take in adequate amounts of food and liquid. **Don't cut back on your dose of insulin or skip any injections. This could lead to significant problems.**

Even if your stomach is upset or your appetite is poor, be sure to take in enough carbohydrate (starch and sugar) to cover your insulin. Try substituting one of the following for each serving of starch, milk, or fruit you normally eat:

1/2 cup apple, orange, grapefruit, or pineapple juice
1/3 cup cranberry juice cocktail, grape juice, or prune juice
3/4 cup regular (not sugar-free) soda pop
2 teaspoon honey
2 1/2 teaspoon sugar
1/3 cup regular (not sugar-free) Jell-O®
6 LifeSavers®
7 jelly beans
1/2 twin Popsicle®

1 slice bread or toast	1 cup soup
6 saltine crackers	1/3 cup tapioca or pudding
1/2 cup hot cereal	1/2 cup eggnog
1/2 cup ice cream	1 cup plain yogurt
1/2 cup sherbet	

In a nutshell, many of the foods you generally avoid when you're well are the ones to eat when you're sick!

"What about food?" Mike asked.

"Well, you know from experience that you may not feel like eating much when you're sick. Even the kinds of foods you want and can tolerate may change."

"So what should I do? I'm taking my insulin and I have to eat something, right?"

"True. Actually, when you're sick you can eat a lot of things that you stay away from when you're well. Here's a list of sick-day foods you should keep handy." (See "Foods for Sick Days," page 77.)

"But I've been told not to eat lots of these things because I have diabetes."

"You noticed that! And of course that's good advice when you're feeling well. But the fact that these foods have a large amount of sugar in a small amount of food is what makes them good choices when you're sick. When you don't feel like eating, you can get enough calories to keep you going and balance your insulin by eating even small amounts of these foods."

"There's sure a lot to know about being sick."

"That's true," the educator agreed. "But it's worth the effort. Doing these things lessens the effect a simple illness can have on your diabetes. And you may save yourself a stay in the hospital."

She then continued through the "When You're Sick" list and discussed the importance of drinking plenty of fluids during an illness. "It's easy to get dehydrated—lose too much water—when you're sick; even easier when you have diabetes, too. You may not drink as much as usual because your stomach is upset. You may lose extra fluids because you're throwing up or because you have diarrhea. And if your blood sugar starts to get high, you'll lose even more water through the urine."

"But what if I'm really sick to my stomach and not able to keep much down?"

"Try swallowing small sips slowly. Take your time. It may take as long as a half hour to get down a half cup of fluid when you're sick. Doing it this way may help to 'sneak it' past an upset stomach. If you try to swallow a full glass all at once, you'll increase the chances of tossing it back up."

"What should I do if I *can't* sneak it past my stomach?" asked Mike.

"I'll have the doctor write you a prescription for a medicine to control nausea and vomiting. I recommend you fill the prescription today so you have the medicine on hand the next time you need it. If you're THAT sick, you won't feel like running out to the pharmacy to pick up supplies."

"That makes sense. Is there anything else I should keep around the house for the next time I get sick?"

"Yes, remember to keep your Glucagon Emergency Kit handy. As we discussed earlier, if you have a low blood sugar reaction and can't keep anything down because of an upset stomach, you can use your Glucagon Emergency Kit to treat a reaction. Then give us a call.

"Also, keep the doctor's and the pharmacy's phone numbers handy. Get a thermometer so you can tell the doctor your temperature. Get some of the items from the "Foods for Sick Days" list. Also lay in a supply of nonprescription medicines that you can use when you're under the weather: things like cough medicine and pain relievers. Some of those products have a good deal of sugar in them, so I'll give you a list of medicines that are sugar-free and safer for you to use." (See page 83.)

"How about testing?" Mike inquired. "Should I test any differently when I'm sick?"

"Blood testing is pretty similar to your normal plan. But because things can change so quickly when you're sick, testing then becomes even more important than when you're well. Do at least four blood sugar tests each day, and test any time you think you might be having a low blood sugar reaction but aren't sure."

"How about urine testing? Is that any different?"

"Yes, it is. When you're sick, we recommend that you do a urine test four times a day, at about the same times that you do your finger-stick blood sugars. In this way, you'll know right away if you start to 'burn the furniture.' If that happens, call the doctor right away so he can help you stay on top of the situation.

"I'd like you to use a double-voided urine sample for the ketone tests you do when you're sick. Then you'll be able to tell if you're still making ketones at the time that you do the test."

"What do you mean by a 'double-voided' urine sample?"

"These are terms we use for urine testing. A single-voided sample contains urine made by the body since the last urination, whenever that might have been. For example, the first urine you pass in the morning is a single-voided sample. If you last urinated before going to bed the night before, the morning urine would consist of urine made all during the night. In order to test a double-voided sample, you would empty your bladder but not test the first sample—the single-voided sample. About a half hour later you would urinate again. This is the sample that you would test. This is called the double-voided sample."

"When would I use each one?"

"The first-voided urine sample in the morning is helpful when you're well. It lets you know how you did during the night. (See "Interpreting Morning Urine Tests for Sugar and Ketones" page 53.). It also alerts you to the presence of any ketones. It's like an early warning system that lets you know if you're having problems. The double-voided urine is helpful when you're sick. Because the urine in a double-voided sample was made during the previous half hour, it tells you how you're doing right at that time. For example, if you test a single-voided urine and find ketones, you don't have any way of knowing exactly when they were made. If it's been six hours since you last urinated, the ketones in the urine sample could have been made at any time during that six-hour period.

"If the ketones were made only during the first hour, it would mean that you're improving. You might need less insulin than if you were still making ketones. A double-voided urine lets you see how you're doing right now. If there are ketones in it, you know that you'll need extra insulin to treat them."

"There's more to this than I ever realized," Mike said. "I can see a lot of things are going to be different the next time I get sick."

Mike left the educator and headed for home. On the way, he stopped at the pharmacy to pick up his sick-day supplies. Then he went to the supermarket and stocked up on Jell-O®, soda pop, and Popsicles®. As he stood in the candy aisle picking out a bag of jelly beans to keep around for sick days, he thought to himself with a smile, "If my other docs could only see me now!"

Sugar-Free
Nonprescription Medicines

Some over-the-counter medicines (such as pain killers, cough medicines, and antacids) contain sugar. The amounts are generally small and may not disturb your diabetes control. But since illness makes it more difficult to control your diabetes anyway, it's best to choose sugar-free varieties when you can.

Use this list to help you choose over-the-counter medications. Read labels before you buy. Avoid those that contain sugar (sucrose, glucose, sorbitol, mannitol, fructose, or dextrose) or alcohol. Read the label every time you buy a product. Manufacturers occasionally change their formulations.

Cough Medicines
(sugar-free, containing little or no alcohol)
> Cerose-DM Liquid
> Colrex Cough Syrup
> Colrex Expectorant Syrup
> Contac Jr. Liquid
> Hytuss Tablets
> Naldecon-DX
> Scot-Tussin Syrup
> Tolused-DM Liquid

Decongestants
> Dimetane Decongestant Elixir
> Dimetapp Elixir
> Novahistine Elixir
> Sinutab Maximum Strength Nighttime Liquid
> Afrin Nasal Spray
> Neo-Synephrine Nose Drops

Pain and Fever Medications (Avoid aspirin. Even though it's sugar-free, large doses can raise the blood sugar.)

Datril
Panadol
Tylenol
Generic acetaminophen
Nuprin
Generic ibuprofen
Children's Panadol (liquid, drops, tablets)
Dolanex Elixir

Sick Day Summary

1. Always take your insulin, even if you can't eat.

2. Keep a supply of sick-day medications on hand.

3. Use Foods for Sick Days when you're too sick to eat your usual meals.

4. Drink plenty of liquids.

5. Take your temperature and record it daily while you're sick.

6. Keep the doctor's and pharmacy's phone numbers handy at all times.

7. Check and record blood sugar and urine ketones at least four times a day while you're sick.

8. Call the doctor if ketones are present.

Section Two

The Flashy Plays

8

The Supermarket Guerilla: More Nutrition

Turkey, lobster, sweet potato pie,
Pancakes piled up till they reach the sky!
                                        —Goofy

Mike paced up and down outside the double doors. He was waiting for the diabetes educator in front of the biggest supermarket in town. When he'd asked her last week how to pick out a cereal that wouldn't send his blood sugar sky high, she'd said it was time for a "tour." It seemed a little silly. After all, he'd been in supermarkets all his life. He hoped he wouldn't see anyone he knew.

He felt a tap on his shoulder. "Am I late, Mike?"

"No. Actually, I was a little early. Gee, Kate, couldn't we do this in the office? I feel a little strange about walking around the supermarket reading food labels."

"If you're really uncomfortable, we can skip it. But if you look around while we're in there, I think you'll see a lot of people reading labels. And they're not all people with diabetes either. Everyone who's trying to watch their weight, cut their risk for heart disease, or just eat a healthy diet needs to know exactly what they're buying. We could do this lesson in the office, but we couldn't do as good a job. Besides, I think seeing and handling the foods will help you remember what we talk about. What do you think?"

"OK, I guess I can take it," Mike replied. "Lead on, general. Where do we start?"

"Funny you should call me 'general,' Mike. One way to think about shopping these days is sort of like a military campaign. There are thousands of possible choices in every supermarket. Tonight's tour is like boot camp. I'm going to make you into a 'supermarket guerilla." You'll be learning to use weapons that will help you defend your blood sugar and your arteries against some other great military leaders: General Mills, General Foods, and Cap'n Crunch®! Let's hit the battlefield."

As Mike and the educator walked into the store, he pulled a grocery cart out of the line-up.

"As long as we're here, I might as well pick up a few things," he explained. "You know, when I first started seeing you, you said to cut down on foods with too much fat and sugar. So I tried reading labels a few times, but I got discouraged. *Everything*'s made with sugar. I can't even find any bread that I like that doesn't have sugar or honey in it."

"Amazing, isn't it?" she commented. "But you've brought up an important point: it's probably not possible to totally avoid sugar. But that's OK, because it's not really necessary to totally avoid it."

Mike picked out a head of lettuce and some tomatoes and put a 10-pound bag of potatoes in the bottom of the cart. "Well, I finally figured out that much. I gave up and bought the whole-wheat bread that had honey in it and nothing drastic happened to my blood sugar. But how do I know where to draw the line? Really sugary things like regular soda pop shoot my blood sugar way up. How much sugar is too much?"

"Well, you're going to hate the answer to that one, Mike: It depends. Let's go down the bread aisle. That's a pretty good place to start.

"You may not know it, but you've already been using one of the supermarket survival weapons I talked about earlier, the ingredients list. We're going to upgrade your use of the ingredients list from the novice to the expert class right now. Do they have the kind of bread you've been buying?"

"Here it is," he replied, "Brannola® Dark Wheat. See, here's the honey on the ingredients list."

"Exactly how far down on the list is it?" she asked.

"It's the sixth item down on the list. Does it make a difference where it is on the list?"

"Yes, a big difference. The list is arranged in decreasing order. The ingredient contained in largest amount is listed first. The ingredient contained in the second largest amount is listed next, and so forth, until we get to the ingredient that there is the least of. It is listed last. So seeing where sugar appears on the list gives you a general idea of how much of it is in the food. The rule of thumb that I use is if sugar isn't one of the first four ingredients, it's probably fine to use the food. Honey is sixth on your bread label, so you made a good choice."

"A keeper for the basket," Mike said as he tossed in two loaves of bread.

"Let's go down this way," the educator suggested. "You were smart to notice the honey. Not everyone pays attention to all the different words for sugary ingredients: sucrose, dextrose, molasses, brown sugar, corn syrup, corn sweeteners, and fruit juice concentrate. They're all just pure sugar."

"So I shouldn't buy foods that have any of those sugar words in the first four ingredients?" he asked.

"That's where the 'it depends' part comes in, Mike. When a food you want has sugar in the first four ingredients, your decision about whether to buy it or not depends on a couple of things. First, think about how much you'll be eating at one time. If it's something that you just use a dab of, like ketchup or sweet pickle relish, it's probably OK. Second, find out if there's another brand of the same item that doesn't contain sugar. Look at these two peanut butter labels. What do you see?"

"Sugar's second on the list in this one," said Mike. "But this one only has peanuts and salt in it. Hey, I like this natural peanut butter better anyway. Another keeper."

"Here's something else, Mike. Tell me what you can about these granola bars."

Mike squinted to read the small print on the label. "Well, corn syrup is third on the list and molasses is fourth. It's even got brown sugar farther down the list. Pretty sweet, huh?"

"Right. Foods that have several sugar ingredients aren't a great choice for everyday use. But here's another 'it depends.' They might be the perfect thing to carry on a long bike ride where you're using up lots of blood sugar exercising.

"There's room for just about any food in a healthy meal plan. To make it work, you just need to figure out how much to use and when. Even regular soda pop has its place. When you're sick, it can help you sneak calories past a queasy stomach, and when you have a reaction, it's easy to find soda just about anywhere."

Rules of Thumb for Identifying High-Sugar Foods

1. Know all the "sugar words:"
   - sugar
   - molasses
   - honey
   - dextrose
   - corn syrup
   - corn syrup solids
   - high fructose corn syrup
   - fruit juice concentrate

2. If a "sugar word" appears AFTER the fourth item in the ingredients list, the food is probably OK.

3. If a "sugar word" is in the first four ingredients, ask yourself:
   - How much will I use at a time? If the amount is very small, like ketchup for example, it's probably OK.
   - Is there another brand of the same thing made without sugar? Example, peanut butter, fruit spreads.

4. If there are several sugary ingredients, question the food's use. Limit use to high energy demand situations like heavy exercise.

"Well, I'm not getting much exercise right now, but I'll keep the granola bars in mind if I get to go skiing this winter. What I AM doing is eating breakfast every day. How do I pick a cereal that doesn't send my blood sugar off the scale?"

"That's what brought us down here in the first place, isn't it? Well, this brings us to the supermarket guerilla's other major weapon: the nutrition information label. I'm sure you've noticed these labels: they show the serving size for the food and the amounts of certain nutrients that you get from a serving that size. Always be sure to check the serving size. Sometimes a really small serving size is shown to make the nutrition information look more acceptable. Here's the cereal section. We couldn't have missed it. I think it's bigger every time I come to the store. Notice that the serving size shown for some really dense cereals like this granola is only one-quarter of a cup. So when you eat a whole bowl full of this, you get about four times as much carbohydrate and calories as for the same volume of a cereal like Cheerios® that has a one-cup serving size."

"So, keeping the size of my cereal serving the same every morning isn't getting the job done?"

"Not unless all the cereals you eat have about the same amount of carbohydrate in a similar size serving. Another thing the cereal nutrition label will tell you is exactly how much sugar is in that serving. It says *Sucrose and other sugars* and lists a number of grams. Here's another rule of thumb for you to remember, if a cereal has 5 or less grams of *Sucrose and other sugars*, you can consider it a low-sugar cereal. Let's check out the cereals you normally buy."

"Most of the time I eat Cheerios, but I also keep Shredded Wheat® and Honey Nut Cheerios® around. Let's see, the Cheerios have a one-cup serving size with 15 grams of carbohydrate and they are low in sugar. I knew those were a keeper because my blood sugar's generally fine after my usual breakfast. But here's one of my problems. Honey Nut Cheerios have more than 5 grams of sugar in a serving and the serving size that give 15 grams of carbohydrate is only *half* a cup. Well, now I know why my blood sugar goes through the roof when I eat these. I get twice as much carbohydrate and sugar in the same size bowl of the Honey Nut kind as I do from the regular Cheerios."

"Would you be happy eating half as much of the Honey Nut kind?"

"No way. I want a full bowl of cereal. I guess I'll have to find another one. I used to like Kix® when I was a kid. Is that one OK?"

Kate handed Mike a box of Kix. "What do you think, Captain? I just gave you a field promotion because you're doing so well."

Picking a Cereal

1. Cereals that have 5 grams or less of "sucrose and other sugars" are "low sugar."

2. To simplify eating a variety of cereals on different days, pick cereals that have about the same serving size and the same amount of carbohydrate per serving. Then eat the same size serving each day.

3. If you want more variety, control serving size to get the right amount of carbohydrate for you. For example, if your insulin is adjusted to cover the 1 1/2 cups of Cheerios (23 grams CHO) you usually eat, you could only eat 1/3 cup of some granola cereals to get the same amount of carbohydrate (unless you learn to adjust your insulin for changing meal size).

4. Whole grain cereals are good choices because of the extra fiber and nutrients they provide.

"The Kix look good. They're low in sugar and the serving size and amount of carbohydrate in a serving is about the same as for my Cheerios. That will give me some variety without shooting my blood sugar into the stratosphere. Oh, that reminds me, what about things that are made with artificial sweeteners? Are they OK for me to eat?"

"Well, sure, Mike. Remember, even regular soda pop has its place but the question is when and how much. Foods that are artificially sweetened fall into two general categories. Things that have very few calories, like Sugar-Free Jell-O, artificially sweetened drink mixes, and diet pop, fall into one group. You can use them in reasonable amounts without much thought. They won't affect your blood sugar much at all.

"But there's another group of artificially sweetened things that is entirely different. Things like hot cocoa mix, sugar-free pudding, and some frozen desserts, including some kinds of frozen yogurt, have ingredients other than the sweetener that have carbohydrates and calories that need to be taken into account. Like Alba Hot Cocoa Mix®. It's sugar-free but has about the same amount of carbohydrates and calories as a piece of bread or a glass of milk."

"I use diet soda all the time," Mike said. "It seems like just about everybody does. But I've never tried sugar-free pudding. I think I'll get some of this to put in my lunches. I can have a cup of pudding instead of a carton of milk with my sandwich and drink a diet soda. Thinking about lunch reminds me, what's the story on low-fat lunch meat? Is that what I should be eating?"

Artificial Sweeteners

1. Find a non-caloric tabletop sweetener you like for use in beverages and on cereal. If you like to bake, find one that's stable in cooking.

2. Read the labels of all artificially sweetened foods. They may have other ingredients that provide calories and carbohydrates that DO affect blood sugar.

3. Artificially sweetened foods that have very few calories, like diet soda, sugar-free gelatins, and low-calorie jellies, can be used freely.

4. Artificially sweetened foods that have calories and carbohydrates must be accounted for in your meal plan. This includes sugar-free hot cocoa mix, frozen yogurt, and pudding.

"In some cases, those lower fat lunch meats can be a pretty good choice, Mike. But when it comes to advertising, remember, 'The large print giveth and the small print taketh away.' Even when the big words on the package look promising, you still need to read the nutrition information label to know exactly what you're getting. Cutting back on saturated fats—the kind you get in meats, dairy products, hydrogenated fats, lard, coconut oil, and palm oil—is one of your most powerful weapons for keeping your blood cholesterol level down.

"A lower fat lunch meat like turkey salami has less animal fat than traditional salami, but it's still not what would be considered a low-fat meat. If you've just got to have salami once in a while, picking the lower fat one makes sense. But there are other sandwich foods that are low in fat and usually less expensive. Sliced turkey breast and boiled ham are both naturally low in fat."

"Are you kidding?" Mike asked. "I thought ham was really high in fat."

"No, ham's actually made from a low-fat pork cut. And it's especially lean when the surface fat has been trimmed away in processing. Look at this Danola® Danish Ham. It's got 35 calories and 1 gram of fat per slice and only 26 percent of its calories come from fat. If you put that on some great crusty rye bread with dark mustard, you've got a very low-fat lunch."

"You know, Kate, that one piece of information made this whole trip worthwhile. Into the basket with the boiled ham. But a little while ago you mentioned a type of oil I should stay away from."

"Yes, Mike. Some of them are definitely better choices than others. The polyunsaturated and monounsaturated fats found in most vegetable oils are better at keeping your heart healthy than the saturated fats found in meat and dairy products. Canola oil, corn oil, safflower oil, and sunflower oil are all good sources of polyunsaturated fats. Use them in cooking and in salad dressing and find a margarine that lists the *liquid* form of one of them as its first ingredient. Monounsaturates are found in olive oil, avocadoes, and nuts. Small amounts of those are fine, too.

"Saturated fats are another matter. Because they play such a big role in raising your blood cholesterol level, I've suggested before that you switch from whole milk to skim or one percent and pick lean cuts of meat. But there are other sources of saturated fat that you need to read labels to avoid. Look out for palm oil, coconut oil, and anything that says 'hydrogenated.' Even though those ingredients might be called 'vegetable' on the label, they're just as hard on your heart as pure lard. They're cheap and they have a long 'shelf life.' Unfortunately, they might shorten *your* shelf life, so try to avoid them. They show up in a lot of processed foods like crackers, cookies, frostings, and snack foods."

"So I'm helping out my heart when I pick these wheat crackers that have liquid safflower oil in the ingredients instead of these cheese flavored ones that say 'partially hydrogenated cottonseed oil and coconut oil'?"

"That's right, Mike. Your basket's getting pretty full."

"You noticed. There's not much room left, actually. Looks like I'm going to eat well this week. One thing I've been wondering about, though. We haven't spent any time in the dietetic food section. Shouldn't I be shopping down there?"

"Well, there may be a few things down there that would be useful to you, Mike. A lot of the people I work with keep sugar-free pancake syrup around and one or two kinds of sugar-free jelly. But don't be fooled by the words 'dietetic' or 'diabetic.' The biggest mistake people make shopping in the diet section is to think that all the foods there are good choices. They're not. You have to be just as careful about reading the labels of dietetic foods as you are of other foods.

"For some items, there may be a better tasting, cheaper version of the same thing in the regular food section that isn't much different nutritionally. Out here in the rest of the supermarket, there are fat-free crackers, low-fat mayonnaise, and salad dressings made with good oil instead of coconut oil. 'Diabetic' cookies, for example, are often sweetened with sorbitol or fructose. While those sugars don't raise blood sugar as quickly as table sugar, they have just as many calories and not everyone likes their flavor. You may find other simple cookies in the regular foods section that you can eat in certain amounts without a problem; for instance, ginger snaps or vanilla wafers.

"Do most of your shopping out where the 'real' foods are, Mike. There's a whole world of good food out there that's good for you: fresh fruits and vegetables; chicken, fish, and lean meat; low-fat and skim-milk dairy products; potatoes, rice, pasta, bread, and cereal. When you eat convenience items like cold cereal, lunch meats, crackers, cookies, snack foods, and bread, read the labels. Know what you're eating. Then you can make good choices to help keep your blood sugar and blood fats under control without having to live on twigs and berries."

Your body's not junk, so why feed it junk food?

9

Joy to the World: Entertaining

Jeremiah was a bullfrog.
He was a good friend of mine.
I never understood a single word he said,
but I helped him drink his wine.

Three Dog Night

"I'm still not sure how I should handle eating out or going to parties," Mike told the educator at his next visit. "Whether I'm going out for fun or for business, I always end up way off my usual schedule. I've had several pretty severe insulin reactions when dinner didn't arrive until after a long cocktail hour.

"I usually take my evening insulin at about a quarter to 6 and eat dinner at 6:30. Most of these things don't even start until 7, and that's just the cocktails. Dinner might not show up until 8 or sometimes even later."

"Changing the time of a meal after you've taken your insulin can create problems," the educator agreed. "Sometimes people who don't have diabetes have a hard time understanding that."

"Yeah, they just think that having diabetes means you can't eat sweets. But at least I've come up with a way to make my friends understand. Now they really listen when I say it's time to get something to eat."

"What do you tell them?"

"Well, I tell them food to me is like air is to a scuba diver. A given amount of air in a tank lasts only so long, and then it's time to get another tank. Then I tell them, 'Pretend you're going diving. Your tank has exactly enough air for one hour. How important would time be to you if you were trapped on the bottom and I promised to bring you a new tank . . . in an hour and ten minutes?'"

"That's a great comparison. Can I use that example with my other patients?"

"Be my guest," Mike replied. "But first help me figure out how to handle my food and insulin when I want to eat out or go to a party."

"Well, I think the troubles you describe are probably related to both delayed meals and to drinking alcohol.

There are ways to handle these situations that should solve your low blood sugar problems," the educator said.

She then went on to explain that there are at least two ways of dealing with delayed meals. One is used when the meal is expected to be only an hour or so later than usual. In that case, simply delaying the time of the insulin injection by an hour will solve the timing problem.

"It's a good idea to add a small snack—a piece of fruit, a glass of milk, or a few crackers—at your usual meal time. Otherwise the insulin from your last shot may drop your blood sugar too low before dinner comes."

"But the delays are usually a lot longer than an hour when I eat out."

"Yes, those 8 or 9 o'clock suppers are an entirely different matter," advised the educator. "We have a different way to manage those.

"When you're expecting a late supper, take your pre-dinner insulin shot at the usual time. Then eat your usual bedtime snack about 30 to 45 minutes later. Depending on the kind of evening you have planned, you might eat the snack before you leave home.

"If there's a cocktail hour, preload a syringe and inject it at the restaurant. Check out the hors d'oeuvres table and order an appetizer. Any combination of crackers, cheese, vegetables, and fruit that approximates your usual bed-time snack will work. Be sure to get about the same amounts of carbohydrate foods—the starches and sugars in bread, fruit, and milk—since this is what will protect you from a low blood sugar reaction. If food isn't available, drink fruit juice or regular soda pop."

"What about dinner?"

"When dinner finally arrives, just stay as close to your normal meal pattern as possible. This whole system works because you're taking in approximately the same total amount of food relative to the same total amount of insulin. It's like depositing your paycheck on the first of the month, but waiting until the fifteenth to pay your bills. The checkbook balance at the end of the month is the same as if you had paid your bills on the first."

"But if I'm going to have a drink during the cocktail hour, shouldn't I decrease the size of my snack? I've got an exchange list for alcohol at home."

"Exchanging alcohol for food is an important concept for people with Type II diabetes, especially those who don't take insulin and are trying to eat fewer calories. The high calorie content of alcohol is their main concern. But when you're taking insulin, especially if you have Type I diabetes, the approach is different.

"Most people don't realize that pure alcohol alone doesn't raise the blood sugar level. In fact, on an empty stomach, it can cause a severe low blood sugar reaction. Remember, the liver is like a factory that produces sugar and then stores it in its warehouse. Insulin causes the factory to decrease production of sugar and to store most of the sugar that it makes. A small amount of sugar, however, is still released into the body at a controlled rate and provides fuel for the body's activities.

"Alcohol shuts down the factory completely and locks the doors on the warehouse. No sugar can be released to the body. So, if you're drinking alcohol and your stomach is empty, your body has no way to get more sugar after it uses up the small amount in the bloodstream. You wind up getting a low blood sugar reaction. That's why it's important to eat if you're going to be drinking alcohol."

"So that's where those reactions have been coming from. I've always reduced the size of my meal when I had a cocktail or two before dinner."

"Well, now you know how to handle it, Mike. But one last thought. If you're going to drink, keep the amounts moderate—no more than one or two drinks a day. More alcohol can really interfere with the control you've been working so hard to establish."

"You know," said the young man, "some of these parties go on for hours. Two drinks won't go very far. But I guess I could switch to diet soda or sparkling water after I reach my limit."

"That's a great idea," she congratulated him. "You know, if your friends are like mine, they're probably so absorbed talking shop or having a good time that they don't really care what you're drinking anyway. The important thing is for you to find a way to have fun without creating a big change in your diabetes control."

Alcohol, Insulin, and Type I Diabetes*

1. If you drink, limit it to two drinks per day.

2. Your best choices are dry wines, light beers, or distilled liquor (i.e., vodka, gin, bourbon, etc.) with noncaloric mixers.

3. Eat your usual amount of food. Drinking on an empty stomach can result in severe low blood sugar reactions.

4. If possible, make sure someone in the group knows you have diabetes and how to treat a low blood sugar reaction.

5. Gasoline and alcohol don't mix. Make sure there's a designated driver in your group.

* If you have Type II diabetes and are overweight, use exchanges to fit alcoholic beverages into your meal plan. If you have Type II diabetes, are normal weight, and take insulin, follow the guidelines given here for Type I diabetes.

10

The Road to Zanzibar: Travel

Out on Runway Number Nine, big 707 set to go,
But I'm stuck here on the grass
where the pavement never grows.

Peter, Paul, and Mary

"Doc," Mike said some weeks later, "I'd like to start planning for my vacation. Do you have any advice?"

"Well, first of all, travel, like the rest of life, can be a lot of fun. But it can also be trying and frustrating.

"As you make your travel plans, keep Murphy's Law in mind: 'Anything that can go wrong, will.' Applied to your vacation, Mike, that means travel is made more fun and less stressful by preparing for any foul-ups that might occur. Planning takes away their power to ruin your good time. The unexpected will still happen—but you'll be ready for it.

"The most important thing to remember is that without your insulin, your vacation would be over. If you break your last bottle of insulin at home, you know exactly where to get some more in a hurry. Away from home, it might not be that simple.

"The bag containing your insulin could be lost or damaged. It could be dropped overboard into the water or fall out of a car or bus. Or it might simply be misplaced. If any of those things happened, you wouldn't want to have all of your eggs in one basket, as they say. A separate bag with a second stash of insulin and syringes would save the day and the trip."

Mike began to see how important it was to bring a back-up supply of insulin on every trip. And he learned to keep all of his insulin in hand-carried bags. Luggage compartments and car trunks can reach temperatures (both too hot and too cold) that can reduce insulin's effectiveness.

"But what if somebody walks off with my carry-on bags?" Mike asked.

"Good for you, Mike. Now you're thinking like Murphy himself! I'll give you prescriptions for your insulin, syringes, and a Glucagon Emergency Kit. Keep them in your wallet or passport case. They could save the day in a real pinch."

"Will I need to change my insulin dose to make a trip?" the young man inquired.

"If you're traveling across more than two time zones, you'll need to adjust the amounts and timing of your insulin doses. When you know your destination and your travel schedule, we can work out a transition plan. It will be based on whether you're traveling east or west and on the time difference between home and your vacation spot."*

"How about if I limit my vacations to places either north or south of here, instead of east or west? Then we wouldn't need to adjust the insulin because of time zone changes."

"Well, that's an idea, isn't it?" chuckled the doctor.

"An idea," Mike agreed, "just not a great one. Wherever I decide to go, I'll probably be going by plane. What can go wrong?"

"Just about everything," the doctor answered. "ASSUME that planes will be late, meals will be absent or delayed, checked luggage will be lost. Carry all the diabetes supplies you might need right on with you.

"Don't check anything you can't afford to be without. But never carry more than you can comfortably schlepp across Chicago-O'Hare at a full gallop when you have only 30 minutes between planes. At the very least, carry insulin,

* See Insulin Adjustments for Time Zone Changes, page 118.

syringes, testing supplies, and enough food to last a day. Carrying glucagon is a good idea, too, especially if you'll be traveling with someone who knows how to use it.

"Remember the air pressure inside of the plane is lower at 35,000 feet than it is when the plane is on the ground. This causes the air inside the insulin bottles to expand. Therefore, you won't need to inject air into the bottle before drawing up your dose if you'll be taking a shot on the plane."

"How about eating on the plane?" Mike asked.

"Airline 'diabetic' meals are sometimes more trouble than they're worth. Some of them look remarkably like a 'regular' meal except for the fact that the flight attendant walks up and down the aisle with yours yelling 'Who's got the diabetic meal?' And occasionally you'll get a thoroughly ridiculous 'super diet' meal that may not have enough calories to cover your normal insulin dose.

"Our educator recommends that you take your chances with the regular meal. Pick and choose from what's on the tray and then use your own food supplies to make that match your normal meal pattern. You can usually count on being able to get both regular and diet soda as well as fruit juice on flights lasting longer than 45 minutes.

"Also, walk around frequently during long flights and drink plenty of liquids. The air is much drier at high altitudes. If you just sit there during the flight, being much less active than usual, your blood sugar may tend to rise. You know from experience that you urinate more when your blood sugar is high. The combination of dry air, a high blood sugar, and frequent urination can really dry you out. If you remember to drink enough liquids and move around occasionally, you'll arrive feeling much more energetic!"

"What if I decide to go on that European vacation you mentioned on the first visit?" asked the young man.

"Sounds great to me," answered the doctor, "but there are a few extra things to keep in mind. Probably the most important is that different types and strengths of insulin are sold in other countries, compared with what you're using here. Since any change in the type, brand, or source of insulin you're using may require you to adjust your doses to maintain blood sugar control, it's best to take extra insulin with you. If you have to change your insulin while on a trip, test your blood sugar more frequently and use Dynamic Insulin Dosing to get the dose corrected as quickly as possible.

"Water supplies and sanitation standards may be different from what you're used to here at home. Exotic 'bugs' in food and water could bother you. If you decide on a trip outside the country, you might find our list of Travel Tips helpful. (See page 120.)

"Once you know what to do about the safety of the food you'll be eating, there's another challenge. You'll need to figure out how the unfamiliar foods being served compare to the meals you usually eat at home.

When you decide on a destination, ask our educator for the food exchange list for the foods of that country. She has lists for several countries. After all, we're not the only place in the world that has people with diabetes."

"But I don't use exchanges. I just keep track of my carbohydrates," Mike explained.

"Even if you're not using an exchange meal plan, you can study the lists to learn about the foods you'll be eating at your destination. The lists can also help you identify appropriate serving sizes and the carbohydrate content of some of the unfamiliar foods.

"Finally, before leaving home, find out how to get medical care on an international trip. One way is to contact the International Association of Medical Assistance to Travelers*.

"If language will be a barrier, be sure to learn at least the phrases you would need to obtain medical care and order appropriate meals. Write those phrases down and keep the paper with you."

* International Association of Medical Assistance to Travelers, 736 Center Street, Lewiston, New York 14092. Telephone (716) 754-4883.

Mike was shaking his head. "All this preparation sounds more like getting ready for a military campaign than heading off on vacation."

"Yes, there really is quite a bit to consider. But if you pay attention to all the details, Mike, you can go anywhere your bank account will allow."

Insulin Adjustments for Time Zone Changes

Adjust your insulin doses and timing when traveling two or more time zones to the east or west. Here are two of the most common ways this type of adjustment can be made.

Option 1.

Switch to a "Basal/Bolus" insulin regimen well before your trip. Basal/Bolus therapy involves taking one or two doses of long-acting insulin to provide a small steady amount of insulin all day and night (the "basal") and a dose of regular insulin about 45 minutes before each meal (a "bolus").

• If traveling West to East, so your day is shortened by three or more hours, decrease the basal, long-acting insulin on the day you travel by 20 percent.

• If traveling East to West so your day is lengthened, add a bolus of Regular insulin for any additional meal(s) eaten on the travel day.

Option 2.

- ### Traveling West to East (day shortened by three or more hours)

One shot per day—Decrease dose by 20 percent on your travel day. Re-establish your regular schedule on the first full day at your destination. Get up on "their" time and proceed with your usual meal and insulin schedule.

Two shots per day—Decrease the second dose by 20 percent. All 20 percent can be taken off the NPH or Lente unless you will be eating a much lighter dinner than usual. In that case, divide the 20 percent reduction between the short-acting and the intermediate-acting insulins. Re-establish your regular schedule on the first day at your destination. Get up on "their" time and proceed with your usual meal and insulin schedule.

- ### Traveling East to West (day lengthened by three or more hours)

One shot per day—Increase your dose by 10 percent on your travel day.

Two shots per day—Add a bolus of regular insulin equal to about 10 to 15 percent of your total daily dose before the extra meal you eat on your travel day.

*If you have Type I diabetes and are taking only one shot each day, talk to your doctor about changing to two or more shots. Type I diabetes cannot be adequately controlled by one shot of insulin per day.

Travel Tips for Extensive Trips

1. If safety of the local water supply is in question:

   • Drink bottled water. Carbonated beverages, beer, and wine in bottles are also safe.
   • Don't use ice cubes.
   • Avoid foods that are washed and served without cooking, such as salad greens or raw fruits. Peeled fruits are OK.
   • Use dental floss to clean your teeth instead of toothpaste and the local tap water.

2. If you are uncertain about the food storage and preparation methods being used:

   • Eat hot foods hot and cold foods cold.
   • Avoid foods containing mayonnaise (refrigeration may be poor).
   • Avoid raw meat and fish (they may carry parasites).
   • Avoid dairy products, including milk and ice cream, unless you know they are pasteurized.

3. Bring an adequate supply of personal toilet articles not always available outside of North America: facial tissues, soft toilet paper, and sanitary napkins.

4. In addition to your insulin and your prescription medication, bring supplies you will need if you should become ill on your trip:

    • medication for nausea and vomiting
    • medication for fever and pain
    • medication for diarrhea
    • a thermometer

5. Bring generous amounts of diabetes supplies:

    • urine strips for glucose and ketones
    • finger-stick blood sugar strips
    • an extra blood glucose meter (repair or replacement may be difficult)
    • extra batteries for your meter
    • syringes

6. Know where to go for medical care. Get this information BEFORE leaving home.

    • If an emergency arises and you cannot reach the health care providers you have identified, contact the nearest U.S. Embassy or Consulate.

When You Travel

1. In a hand-carried bag, pack:

   - At least one day's supply of food
   - Insulin and syringes
   - Glucagon
   - Glucose meter, strips, and lancets
   - Urine ketone test strips
   - Prescriptions
   - Other medications you use
   - List of medical facilities at your destination

2. Take a backup supply of critical items, packed in a separate bag.

3. When crossing time zones, work out a transition plan for insulin with your doctor.

4. Before leaving home, prepare a plan for obtaining emergency medical care while you're away.

11

Up Off the Couch! Exercise

Let's get physical. . .
—Olivia Newton-John

"You know, Doc," the young man observed, "there's something else I'd like to learn about—exercise. I love to run and play tennis, but I've had so many low blood sugar problems when I exercised in the past that it didn't seem worth the trouble. It took all the fun out of it for me."

"Well, if it's not fun you probably won't do it. So let's see what we can do.

"First, it's great that you love to exercise. But, you know, there are some other good reasons to exercise BESIDES fun.

"People who exercise regularly have a greater sense of well-being and are better able to deal with stress. Their energy level is higher, and their stamina is greater. Exercise even helps to lower blood pressure, control weight, and decrease the risk for heart disease. In fact, doctors have been recommending exercise for people with diabetes since about 600 B.C."

"I've heard all that before, Doc, but are the benefits worth the risk of a low blood sugar?"

"Yes, I think they are. And I'm not the only one who thinks that. There's even an organization whose sole purpose is to encourage people with diabetes to be more active. It's the IDAA* and I'd suggest you join up. You might get some helpful ideas from meeting other active people with diabetes."

"But I'm no athlete, Doc."

"That's OK, Mike. IDAA members run the gamut from people who do triathalons to those whose most strenuous activity is jumping to conclusions. Every level of sport and recreation is encouraged. But no matter what your level of activity is going to be, you need to prepare. When you do, you greatly reduce the risk of reactions and other problems. There are a few things you need to learn."

"So teach me! That's why I'm here."

*International Diabetic Athletes Association, 1931 E. Rovey Avenue, Phoenix, AZ. Phone (602) 230-8155. Yearly dues - $12.

"Well, the first step is picking your sport," the doctor said.

"Actually, I'd like to go back to jogging."

"That's a good choice for you. You don't have any joint or foot problems that might be stirred up by running. For people who do have those difficulties, walking or swimming would be a better way to get started. But now that you've picked your sport, let's prepare for it. I recommend that you start by getting good, well-fitting footwear as well as good, well-fitting diabetes gear."

"Well-fitting diabetes gear?"

"Yes. For example, a diabetes ID of some type, like a bracelet or necklace, would be helpful. It can alert other people to get the right kind of help if you should have a problem while you're exercising. And having a Glucagon Emergency Kit along with other items to treat or prevent low blood sugars such as juice, crackers, or glucose gel is also important. Of course, if you're planning long workouts, you'll need a supply of water. And it's best to have blood sugar testing materials with you as well."

"Are you sure you're not sending me out for an overnight camping trip, Doc? Where am I supposed to put all this stuff? I'd need to borrow the side-car off my brother's motorcycle."

"It's not that bad, Mike," the doctor laughed. "It will all fit in the same athletic bag you carry your sweats or shoes in. Most people just set the bag down in the area where they're working out."

"But how about when I run? If I'm two miles out and start to have a reaction, I'm not going to be able to make it back to some bag."

"For a moving exercise like running or biking, use a 'runner's belt.' They're big enough to hold what you'll need."

"My meter won't fit in one of those. And I wouldn't want something that heavy jarring against me when I run anyway. I suppose I could just carry visually read strips and lancets. That's the way I tested my blood before I got my meter."

"That's one solution," the doctor agreed. "Another possibility is to use one of the smaller meters. Some are no larger than a ball point pen or even a credit card. Remember, well-fitting gear gets the job done."

"I understand this is all stuff I'd need if something went wrong. But what I really want to know is how to prevent problems in the first place."

"Thinking like Murphy again! You're OK," the doctor complimented him. "I was just getting to that. The first way to avoid trouble is to make sure your diabetes is in good control before you begin to exercise."

"I know that. I always check my blood sugar before any kind of workout. If it's high, I skip the exercise."

"Do you also check for ketones before you exercise?" the doctor asked.

"Ketones? No. Why?"

"Because a high blood sugar by itself may not necessarily be a reason to cancel a workout," the doctor answered.

"Really? My last doc told me never to exercise if my blood sugar was over 250."

"That's pretty common advice, but it misses the point. If you're feeling good and don't have ketones in your urine, you can exercise at that blood sugar level. However, if you do have ketones, that's very important information. It tells us that your body won't respond well to exercise."

"How can that be?"

"Think of the log cabin. When you have ketones in your urine, you're 'burning the furniture' instead of the wood from the woodpile. When that happens, you need to find out what the problem is and correct it before you begin to exercise. Otherwise, the exercise is just going to make matters worse."

"I don't understand."

"Remember, when you're 'burning the furniture,' your body is using fat rather than sugar for energy because it can't get sugar into the cell. This happens when there isn't enough insulin around to open the door. It can also happen when there just isn't enough blood sugar around—like when you're having an insulin reaction.

"Since exercise increases your need for energy, exercising when you have ketones makes you 'burn the furniture' at an even faster rate. Continuing to exercise will just increase your level of ketones. As the level rises, you'll begin to feel weak and tired. In an extreme situation, all those ketones could even cause you to go into DKA (diabetic ketoacidosis)."

"So, obviously, exercising when I have ketones wouldn't be smart," Mike said. "What should I do?"

"If you find ketones when you get up in the morning and your blood sugar is in the normal or low range, test for ketones again a couple of hours after breakfast. If the ketones are gone by then, they were probably caused by a low blood sugar reaction during the night. You could go ahead with your exercise.

"If, instead, when you wake up, you find ketones and a fairly high blood sugar, say over 250, you have a real problem. Switch to your sick day schedule and skip your workouts. When your diabetes is back under control you can go back to your normal workouts."

"But won't I get out of shape if I miss a workout?"

"No, Mike, you don't need to exercise everyday in order to stay in shape. In fact, when you exercise with ketones in the urine, you're actually tearing down muscle rather than building it up."

"Well, I don't want to do that. Will the same thing happen if I have high sugars and no ketones?"

"No, as long as there are no ketones in your urine and you feel good, go ahead and exercise. If you don't feel good, skip it. And don't fall into the trap of feeling you *have* to exercise to bring down a high blood sugar."

"What do you mean?"

"Exercise for fun. Exercise for relaxation. Exercise for health. And understand how exercise affects your blood sugar. But use all the other tools we've talked about to keep your blood sugars where you want them to be.

"Right now, though, your main concern is low blood sugar reactions during exercise. So let me explain how exercise decreases your need for insulin.

"Let's go back to the log cabin again. If a stiff breeze began to blow through the open door, fanning the flames in the fireplace, the fire would burn much faster than before. You would have to feed logs to the fire at a faster rate. Exercise is like the stiff breeze. It causes you to burn fuel faster and decreases your need for insulin."

"How much less insulin will I need?" Mike asked.

"That depends on how long and how hard you exercise. By checking your blood sugar before and after exercise, you can figure out how much to decrease the insulin. The reduction might be as little as 10 percent for a one-hour run or as much as an 80 or 90 percent drop if you were going to run a marathon.

"If you do about the same amount of activity at about the same time every day, you can adjust your usual insulin doses to that routine. But if the time you work out changes from day to day, it's tricky to make accurate insulin adjustments. Therefore, if possible, I recommend exercising at the same general time every day."

"When I was running regularly, it was nearly always in the morning," Mike said. "I'll probably do the same again. But how about the times when I haven't planned to exercise? My girlfriend and I like to play tennis. But I usually don't know until the afternoon if we're going to play that day or not."

"You can't take away insulin that was injected earlier in the day when you decide to exercise on the spur of the moment. But you *can* adjust the amount of food that's available. Eat an extra serving of fruit or starch for each 30 to 45 minutes of moderate exercise. You'll do better if you do this before and during exercise to PREVENT a reaction instead of waiting to feel symptoms and then treating them."

"Sounds great. What kind of fruit or starch would you recommend?"

"Apples, bananas, and grapes should work. Try whatever you enjoy that agrees with you when you're active. A half dozen soda crackers, a small box of raisins or a small can of orange juice should also work well and are pretty easy to carry. If your workout is going to be really hard or lengthy or if the weather's hot, concentrate on juices or soft fruits that provide fluids along with the carbohydrates.

"Is there anything else I need to do?" Mike was anxious to get started.

"Yes, as a matter of fact, there are two more things to be aware of. One is to make sure you get enough fluids when you exercise. If you lose too much water—get 'dehydrated'—your performance will suffer. It can also disturb your diabetes control. Drink while you're exercising. Don't wait to get thirsty. About 4 to 8 ounces of fluid for each 15 minutes in your workout should keep you in good shape.

"The last thing is to make sure you get enough food—not only before and during your workout, but after it, too."

"What do you mean?" Mike asked.

"When you exercise for very long, your body uses up emergency sugar supplies stored in the muscles and liver. It will replace these stores later on, after you've finished exercising. Your blood sugar is likely to drop quite a bit when that happens. And if you exercise late in the day, that blood sugar drop could happen during the night. So it's important to continue to check your blood sugar AFTER long workouts. You may need an extra snack to prevent that drop in blood sugar.

"A long workout is sort of like taking out a loan from the bank. At some point, you'll have to pay back the extra energy you used. Make sure your body has something around to pay that blood sugar 'bill' when it comes due."

Getting Set to Exercise

Before you get started . . .

1. Wear a diabetes ID that shows your name, address, phone number, person to contact in an emergency, and your doctor's name and phone number.

2. Get well-fitting athletic shoes that protect and support your feet. If you have trouble getting a good fit, see a podiatrist or orthopedic specialist.

3. Get a Glucagon Emergency Kit. Teach your exercise partner(s) how and when to use it.

4. Get a "runner's belt" to carry diabetes supplies.

What to take with you when you exercise:

1. Things to prevent and treat low blood sugar:
   - Glucose gel or tablets
   - Candy
   - Fruit juice or sport drink
   - Fruit or crackers

2. Diabetes ID

3. Glucagon Emergency Kit

For long workouts, also carry . . .

1. Water, if not available where you'll be exercising.

2. Blood testing supplies.

During exercise . . .

1. Check blood sugar and urine ketones before you begin.

2. Schedule workouts for the same time each day, if possible.

3. Drink plenty of fluids.

4. Eat enough food to fuel activity and cover your insulin.

5. Eat a serving of fruit or starch every 30 to 45 minutes of activity.

6. Learn to reduce your insulin appropriately for hard or lengthy exercise. Having too much insulin acting during exercise creates a high risk for low blood sugar reactions.

12

The Gown Opens
in the Back!
And Other Hazards of
Same-Day Surgery

When nothin' I do
don't seem to work,
It only seems to make matters worse
On me...
Here comes your 19th nervous breakdown
—The Rolling Stones

As Mike drove home from work, he turned up the radio to hear the weekend weather forecast. "Good news for you skiers," the weatherman reported. "There's a 70 percent chance of more snow this weekend to top off the heavy storms of the last week. All lifts should be open."

"Great!" Mike thought to himself. "It seems like I've been waiting forever for the new ski season to start. I'll start getting my gear together tonight and head up to the mountains this weekend."

His ski jacket and pants were easy to find because they were hanging in the back of the closet right where he'd put them last spring. A little searching turned up his hat, gloves, and long underwear on a back shelf. And his ski socks finally emerged from under the swimsuits and tennis clothes in the bottom drawer of his dresser. Mike poked his finger through a hole in the bottom of one of the socks.

"Guess I need to buy some new socks. I hope the rest of my gear is in better shape."

Now to get his skis and other equipment. Mike knew they were stored out of the way, up in the attic. He pulled the attic stairs down out of the ceiling. As he reached the top of the rickety ladder, he saw the skis leaning against the far wall, next to the poles and boots. The goggles were on a nearby shelf. "It looks like everything's in one piece," Mike thought.

Plopping the goggles on his head, he put the skis under one arm and pinned the poles to his body with the other. Then he grabbed the boots and headed for the ladder. Snow covered slopes filled his mind as he carefully juggled the load. "Why make two trips when one will get the job done?" He twisted to fit the tips of the skis through the stair opening and started down.

Unfortunately, Mike was jerked to a stop on the third step when his sleeve caught on a nail. The poles shifted as his upper body was pulled back and the skis began to slip. He dropped the boots in an effort to stop his fall, but it was too late. Mike and all his ski gear clattered down the stairs, landing in a tangled pile on the floor. When the crashing and banging was over, Mike could tell he had a real problem. His right knee was throbbing. He'd twisted it badly in the fall.

"I can't believe I banged myself up before I even made it to the mountain. I'm going to take a lot of ribbing over this one."

Leaving the ski gear where it fell, Mike hobbled into the kitchen and made up an ice bag for his knee. He spent the rest of the night propped up on the couch watching TV.

The next morning, the knee was still stiff and swollen. "I must have really injured it," Mike decided. "I think I'd better make an appointment with that orthopedic surgeon I saw last year." He'd helped Mike a lot when he injured his ankle playing basketball.

Late that afternoon, Mike winced with pain as the doctor probed the puffy knee. "I think you might have a torn ligament, Mike, but I want to be sure. Take it easy on the knee and come back in two weeks for a recheck. The knee should be easier to examine by then." He wrote prescriptions for pain medication and crutches. Mike thanked him and hobbled out of the office.

Two weeks later, on re-examination, the orthopedic surgeon confirmed his fears. "I'm afraid there is a torn ligament, Mike. I recommend arthroscopy to get you back in shape."

"What's that, Doc?" Mike asked.

"It's a type of surgery. Instead of making a big incision to open up your knee, I'll use an instrument that's like a small telescope. I'll only have to make a small cut in the skin of the knee to place it inside. It lets me examine the knee from the inside and repair it without making a large incision. You'll heal up a lot faster than you would after standard knee surgery."

"That doesn't sound too bad. Is there anything special that I need to do to get ready for this?"

"Just a few simple things, Mike. We'll do the procedure at the outpatient surgical center as same-day surgery. You'll come in, have the operation, and go home all in the same day. My nurse will give you a sheet of instructions to help you get ready."

"Will my diabetes be a problem?"

"No, Mike, don't worry. We do this all the time with diabetic patients. Trust me. Just follow the instructions and you'll do fine."

The nurse arranged a date for the surgery and gave Mike an instruction sheet. It contained a few simple instructions. "Don't eat anything after midnight on the night before your operation. Take half your usual insulin dose on the morning of surgery. Report to the outpatient surgical center at noon. Your operation will be at 2 PM. You can go home at about 5."

On the morning of surgery, a hungry Mike took half of his usual dose of insulin and drove to the outpatient surgical center. As he was checking in, he began to feel lightheaded and broke into a sweat. "I must be more nervous about this than I thought," he told himself. But as the feeling got worse, he realized he was having a low blood sugar reaction.

He hadn't eaten anything since his snack the night before, so there was no food in his stomach to counteract the insulin he'd taken earlier that morning. He could tell he was heading for trouble. He knew he should eat to treat the reaction, but he wasn't supposed to eat because of the surgery. He froze. He didn't know what to do. He panicked.

The next thing Mike knew, he was lying on the floor with a nurse kneeling next to him. "Welcome back," she said. "I gave you a shot of glucagon. Now that you're awake, I'd like you to drink this juice and eat a few crackers. You'll feel better in a few minutes."

Mike felt terrible. But as the glucagon and juice had their effect, he began to feel more normal.

A tall woman in green surgical scrubs walked over to where Mike was sitting. "Are you feeling better?" she asked.

"Not bad," Mike replied. "Can I go in for my surgery now?"

"I'm afraid not, Mike. I'm Dr. Shapiro. I was supposed to be the anesthesiologist for your operation, but now that you've had to eat something to treat that reaction, I can't put you under with anesthesia. It wouldn't be safe. You'll need to reschedule your surgery."

"Why wouldn't it be safe? I'm feeling a lot better. Honest."

"I'm glad to hear that, but the safety problem doesn't have anything to do with how you feel but rather with what's in your stomach. It's best to give you anesthesia on an empty stomach. Sometimes anesthesia can make your stomach feel queasy and cause you to throw up. If you've eaten and this occurs, you might choke on pieces of food or suck them into your lungs. So we need to reschedule this to another day when your stomach is empty."

Mike was feeling awful again, but this time it didn't have anything to do with his blood sugar level. He had planned the surgery around his work schedule, now he'd have to juggle his appointments again. His boss wouldn't be happy.

When Mike returned to work the next day, he decided to deal with the situation head-on. He told his boss what had happened.

"You must be disappointed, Mike. I know you really need to get that knee taken care of," his boss said. "But aren't you going to just have another reaction if you do the same thing next week?"

"That occurred to me too, so I'm going to see the doctor who takes care of my diabetes tomorrow. Maybe he can come up with a better plan."

The next day Mike's doctor shook his head as the young man described what had happened to him at the surgical center. "It's a shame you had so many problems, Mike. But with the insurance companies and the government trying to control health care costs, same-day surgery centers and shortened hospital stays are being used much more. Because of this, problems just like you describe are occurring a lot more often than they used to. What happened to you is absolutely predictable and expected for a person with Type I diabetes."

"Well, why didn't the surgeon know that? He said he takes care of people with diabetes all the time and never has problems."

"I'm sure it just didn't occur to him, Mike. Remember, 80 to 90 percent of the people who have diabetes have Type II. People with Type II diabetes can go for a longer period of time without food than people like you with Type I diabetes. So they don't usually get in trouble when they don't eat anything after midnight in preparation for surgery. And because doctors and nurses successfully treat so many patients with Type II diabetes, they may tell you 'Don't worry, we do this all the time. Your diabetes will be fine.' They might not realize the difference between Type I and Type II diabetes.

"Your situation with Type I diabetes is very different from that of a person who has Type II diabetes. You need to be prepared for surgery in a very different way. We've actually had a couple of patients with Type I diabetes develop severe reactions while they were driving to the hospital for surgery. At least you were somewhere where you could get help when you went down for the count."

"Yeah, I guess it could have been worse. But what about next week? How do I stop it from happening again? Would it help if I took even less insulin on the morning of the surgery?"

"No, that's not the answer, Mike. Remember, you need insulin just like you need air and water. You don't breathe less air when you're getting ready for surgery, do you? If you tried it, you'd get short of breath. It's the same thing with your insulin. By taking less insulin than you really need, you run the risk of developing diabetic ketoacidosis. Without enough insulin to hold the doors of the cells open, you'll have to 'burn the furniture' in order to survive. You don't need those kind of problems on top of the stress of surgery."

"So you're saying that I should take my usual dose of insulin on the morning of surgery. But how can I do that? I passed out cold when I only took half my usual dose."

"Mike, what we need to do is admit you to the hospital on the day before your surgery in order to get you properly prepared."

"I'm scheduled to work that day. Don't tell me I have to take another day off from work."

"No, Mike. We'll admit you right after supper so you won't have to miss any more work."

"But the hospital is going to cost more than the outpatient surgical center. Will my insurance allow that?"

"Your insurance company might say no at first. If they do, I'll explain to them that you need to be admitted because you have Type I, not Type II, diabetes. I've never had a problem with an insurance company once I've explained the situation to them. They allow the admission because they realize the severe problems that you can get into with Type I diabetes when preparing for surgery. We'll call them tomorrow and get the approval process started."

"What can you do differently in the hospital to prepare me for the surgery?"

"We'll put an IV (intravenous) line in the vein in your arm and run sugar water through it. That will give you the calories you need to balance your insulin while you're not eating. And I'll have the nurses do finger-stick blood sugars every few hours to make sure your blood sugar is staying in a safe range. If your sugar gets too low, we'll just increase the rate of the IV to let more sugar water run into your body. If your sugar gets too high, we'll decrease the rate. But either way, we'll have control."

"That makes a lot of sense. Things should go a lot better next week when we try it again. But let me ask you this. Does this mean that anytime I'm told not to eat anything after midnight that I'll need to be admitted to the hospital?"

"Yes, Mike, that's right. It's the best way to control your diabetes in that situation. In fact, *whenever* anyone tells you not to eat anything after midnight—whether it's for surgery or even a test—that should immediately raise a red warning flag with you. Tell the doctor, nurse, or technician that you have Type I diabetes and explain what we've just talked about."

"Give me an example, Doc."

"Well, for instance, a study called an 'upper GI' is done to check people for a stomach ulcer. With this test, you swallow a substance that lines the stomach and makes any ulcers show up better on the X-ray. If there were food in the stomach, it might block the view of the stomach wall. So you'd be told not to eat after midnight in preparation for the test. For all the reasons we just discussed, it would be best to bring you into the hospital the night before. Then we could keep your diabetes under control while the test was being done.

"Another thing to remember, Mike, since we're on the subject, is that some tests involve extended preparation. For example, when X-rays are taken of the lower bowel, patients have to take medicine to clean out the bowel and drink nothing but liquids for the whole day before the X-ray is taken. This is called a bowel prep. Done in the normal way, a bowel prep would put you at great risk of having a low blood sugar reaction because the stomach and the bowel are empty."

"What would I do in that situation, Doc?"

"If you had Type II diabetes, Mike, you could do the bowel prep at home. We'd change your insulin dose a bit. You'd do fine. But because you have Type I diabetes, I'd strongly recommend that you be admitted to the hospital for the bowel prep and X-ray. We'd set up an IV line running sugar water into your arm. There would be plenty of sugar on board and you could have the prep and the test done without risking a serious low blood sugar reaction."

"Boy, it's really difficult when you have diabetes."

"Mike, I know it takes more time and money to do these things but it only becomes a *problem* if you don't take the proper precautions. When you prepare in advance, things can go very smoothly and you can do quite well. Which leads me to one last item, your schedule. I'm going to ask your surgeon to schedule the surgery for early in the morning. That will make it much easier to manage your diabetes. We'll have time to wait until after the anesthesia has worn off to make sure you can eat without any vomiting. Then we'll send you home. I don't want you having a reaction at home after we discharge you."

Mike's doctor called the orthopedic surgeon and arranged for the admission to the hospital on the night before Mike's surgery. His case would be the first one of the day. Mike left the office still feeling pain in his knee but at least feeling relieved that his diabetes would be under control all during the surgery.

This time there were no surprises. Mike drove himself to the hospital on the evening before his surgery. The IV was started and the nurses began checking his blood sugar every few hours. He woke up in the morning feeling fine and got his morning dose of insulin. At 7:30 AM, a nurse came to his room with a wheelchair. Mike climbed in and was rolled down to the operating room. He really felt confident because everything was going well. No reactions. No delays. No problems.

"Hi, Mike. How are you?" Mike recognized the anesthesiologist behind her surgical mask.

"Fine, Dr. Shapiro. A lot better than the last time we met."

"I'm glad to hear it, Mike. It's amazing how much difference a little planning and a bottle full of sugar water can make."

"All the difference in the world." It was the surgeon. "Well, Mike, are you ready for surgery?"

"What's to get ready, Doc? I just provide the body!"

They all laughed because now they knew better.

**Withholding food or insulin
in Type I diabetes
can be dangerous.**

**For this reason,
many diagnostic tests
and even minor surgical
procedures are best
handled in the hospital.**

Section Three

And Other Things

13

Morley Safer's in the Waiting Room: Stress

I would not be convicted by a jury of my peers,
still crazy after all these years.

—Paul Simon

The educator was reviewing Mike's blood sugar records at one of his regular visits. She noticed a definite change in blood sugar patterns toward the end of each month.

"If you were a woman, I'd have a good idea of what's going on," she remarked. "For a lot of women, hormone changes during the menstrual cycle cause blood sugars to go out of control in a fairly predictable fashion. Changes in the insulin dose can usually compensate for that. But that obviously can't be your problem, Mike. What's up?"

"I've noticed that myself," the young man replied. "The only thing I can think of is that I work longer hours toward the end of each month. I have to complete all of my end-of-the-month paper work."

"Maybe stress is affecting your blood sugar."

"Stress. . . .You may be right," he replied. "Especially when I'm waiting for the monthly sales figures to come in. My commission check depends on meeting those sales quotas."

"Well, I think we may have our answer," she agreed and went on to describe how stress can disturb blood sugar control. She used Mike's hectic month-end schedule to illustrate her point. "With extra demands on your time and your concentration, stress can affect your blood sugar by changing your routine. When you're feeling stressed, you may not be as careful about eating and taking your insulin on time. Or maybe you eat differently because you're rushed and don't take the time to prepare your usual meals.

"Some people use more sweets and alcohol to cope during stressful periods. You might even get careless about how much insulin you're drawing up because you're worried about what the boss is going to think of your report. In short, there are a lot of ways feeling stressed can directly affect the way you manage your diabetes."

"I can see that, and I'm sure that was happening at first," Mike said. "But recently I've been more careful about food and insulin. Even so, the blood sugars are still a little higher and more erratic during the last week of each month than they are at other times."

The educator then described another way feeling stressed can affect blood sugar.

She explained that when we see life events as threats or "stressors," the body produces the so-called "stress" hormones. These hormones make fuel—sugar—available in case you need to fight or run away. That was a great response when most threats were physical—a saber-toothed tiger waiting in the bushes or a neighboring tribesman charging up behind you with a club.

"Most of the things people think of as being stressful these days—a tough supervisor, a grouchy neighbor, or stop-and-go traffic—can't be dealt with in physical terms," the educator continued. "And so the extra sugar freed up by the stress response goes unused. When this happens in a person with diabetes, the usual insulin dose just can't keep things in line. The result can be high or erratic blood sugars.

"Stress is an everyday part of everyone's life. Even good things like getting a promotion or buying a beautiful new car can be stressful. In fact, being ALIVE means you'll have stress. But it's how we respond to changes and challenges that actually determines our level of stress. 'Stressors' are usually external events, although our own thoughts can certainly be stress-inducing, but 'stress' itself is always an entirely INTERNAL event."

The educator used a story to illustrate.

It's Friday night in Hoboken. Old Overshoe Airlines has the last flight of the evening to Chicago. The plane is an hour late and at least 50 percent overbooked. After the ticket agents calm down most of the crowd by giving them free tickets, two sales people are left standing at the gate: Joan B. Cool and Frank Lee Steamed.

When informed she won't be able to get out of town until the "red eye" flight at 1 AM, Joan thanks the attendant, calls her husband and sits down in the departure lounge with a new adventure novel. "I haven't had five minutes to spare all week," she says to herself. "I could use some time to myself."

Frank Lee Steamed, on the other hand, makes a loud and detailed commentary on the ticket agent's IQ and threatens never to fly Old Overshoe again. He spends the next four hours telling everyone within earshot how badly he's been treated while he pops down aspirin and antacid tablets.

Frank is definitely having a stress reaction! But Joan calmly accepts the change in plans. She even uses the extra time to relax and enjoy herself. The external event is the same. It's what Joan and Frank are saying to themselves about it that makes the event stressful or not.

"The message," said the educator, "is that things that can lead to stress are bound to happen. When they do, your diabetes control may be affected. Everybody has stress, but you can reduce its effect on your life. Take a calm look at the situation. Try to see it in a positive light. ACT on your stressors, instead of letting them act on you."

Stress

1. RECOGNIZE when you're under stress.
2. IDENTIFY what you're saying to yourself that makes events in your life seem more stressful.
3. WHENEVER possible, "reframe" your thinking to view things in a positive light.
4. COMMUNICATE your feelings to people who add to your stress. Be assertive.
5. ACT to meet the challenge. Plan your time. Manage your work load. Learn to say NO.
6. MINIMIZE the effects of stress:
   - Approach life with a sense of humor— LAUGH!
   - Take control of your own life.
   - Make life more meaningful by seeking a satisfying role in family, work, and community.
   - Approach life with enthusiasm, seeing change as a challenge or opportunity.
   - Relax without guilt. Make time for leisure. Smell the roses.
   - Eat healthful foods and exercise regularly.
   - Get enough sleep.
   - Limit or eliminate alcohol.
   - Abstain from using tobacco and other forms of substance abuse.
   - Develop inner peace by identifying your own values and acting on them.
   - Learn to use some form of relaxation, such as deep breathing or yoga.

14

That'll be $378.92: Reimbursement and Coverage for Diabetes Care

Just give me money. That's what I want!
—The Beatles

One day Mike stopped to read a bright poster on the bulletin board at work. The words "Choose your Health Plan" had caught his eye. The annual period for open enrollment in the four health insurance plans offered by his company was coming up. Mike knew that his diabetes made choosing the right insurance plan very important. He decided to learn as much as he could this time before making his choice.

He called the personnel office and made an appointment with the benefits manager. Even after reading the pamphlets for each insurance plan, there was still a lot he didn't understand. He hoped the benefits manager would be able to clear things up for him.

On the morning of the appointment, he walked into her office with a list of questions in one hand and his past year's medical bills in the other.

"Hi, Mike. I'm Carrie MacGuire. I understand you have some questions about the open enrollment period."

"Hi, Carrie. Thanks for seeing me. Actually my questions aren't so much about the enrollment period as about how to make a good choice. I want to get the right coverage, but I don't want to pay any more than I have to."

"I'm glad to see someone taking the decision seriously, Mike. Health care coverage is expensive. But it's not nearly as expensive as being without it or having the wrong kind if you have a major health problem. What exactly did you want to know?"

Mike explained that he had two big concerns. One of them was whether his diabetes would keep him from being accepted by whatever new plan he chose. The other was how to pick the plan that gave him the best coverage for the services he needed.

"I'm in great health, Carrie. But to stay that way, I have regular visits with my doctor and diabetes educator, periodic lab work, and the ongoing costs of medicine, blood testing supplies, and other things. It's pretty expensive. I want a plan that helps me *stay* healthy by paying for some or all of that care. I don't want one that waits until I'm in bad shape before it kicks in. That's not smart with diabetes."

"As far as being able to switch plans, Mike, that's always a concern when you have an existing medical condition. But it's less of a problem with group insurance like you have here at work. The idea of insurance is to spread the risk of developing an illness, injury, or disease among a lot of people.

"When you're insured as part of a group, the amount you pay for a given level of insurance coverage—the premium—is lower than it would be if you bought the same amount of insurance on your own. That's because the risk is spread across all members of the group.

"In a big group, a lot of people will stay healthy and require very few medical services. They balance off the risk that the insurance company is taking by guaranteeing to pay for everyone's expenses. So group insurance is generally a good choice for people who have an ongoing condition like yours, Mike. It's cheaper. It's also less likely to be cancelled because a few people have major medical bills. If you have major claims with insurance that you hold individually, you run a pretty high risk of having your policy cancelled."

"I know about the value of good group health insurance," Mike said. "It was a big factor when I was looking for a job. I can't imagine what people with diabetes do if they can't get insurance at work."

"Well, there are some options," Carrie replied. "People who work for small companies and those who are self-employed may be eligible for insurance plans sponsored by their churches or clubs, by unions and trade groups, or even alumni associations. But wherever you get your insurance, be careful when you change plans. Never let one insurance plan lapse until you've received written notice of being accepted by the new insurer. Some people call going without insurance 'going naked.' And naked is not a good way to be with health care costs at an all time high."

"How long do I have to keep the old insurance going after I've applied for the new one?" Mike asked.

"Most companies take about thirty days to deliver the new policy. But be patient. Don't cancel your old policy until you actually receive written approval from the new plan."

"I'll remember that," said Mike. "I made a list of all the health care services I've used during the last year. I'd like to compare it with the coverage provided by each of the plans you're offering. I figure that knowing what they'll pay for and what I'll have to pay for will help me pick the best plan."

"That will take some time," Carrie said, "but it's the best way I know to make a good choice. I'll get you the Schedule of Benefits and rate sheet for each plan. Besides looking at what is and isn't covered, also figure out what your out-of-pocket expenses are likely to be with each plan. That's not just the premium. It's also any charges the insurance company *won't* pay and the deductible. The deductible is the amount of covered expenses that you have to pay yourself each year before the insurance company begins to pay. One plan has a $250 deductible, two are $500, and one is $1,000. Generally, the lower the deductible, the higher the premium.

"You'll also want to keep track of how much you'll have to pay AFTER you've met the deductible for the year. Depending on the policy, that's called either the co-payment or the co-insurance. For a couple of the plans, the co-insurance is a percentage of each bill—say 20 percent. That means the insurance company pays 80 percent of a covered expense and you pay the other 20 percent. For the other plans, there are specific co-payments set for certain items: $5 for a prescription, $10 for an office visit, and so on. The insurance company pays the difference between the bill and your co-payment.

"You're trying to make a risk management decision. In risk management, you want to balance an acceptable loss (what you pay for premiums, deductibles, co-payments, and uncovered expenses) against an acceptable gain (what the insurance company pays for the services you need). Look for a plan that will return about 65 to 75 percent of your health insurance premiums as benefits. That's considered a fair benefit return."

"I think I'm going to need my calculator for this one," Mike said. "But I'm interested in more than just cost. There are a couple of other things that I'm wondering about, too. For instance, can changing plans affect where I get my care?"

"Oh, good question, Mike. It sure can. Is choosing your doctor important to you?"

"I can't tell you how important. It took me a long time to find the right doctor and I just won't change," Mike answered.

Carrie smiled. "Well, you just eliminated one of the choices. Our HMO (health maintenance organization) is a Staff Model HMO. That means it employs its own medical staff. It doesn't pay anything toward services provided by a doctor from outside the plan. If staying with your current doctor is that high a priority, you need to look at the other plans instead. It's too bad, though, our HMO is the cheapest plan."

"Well, cheap is great, but getting the right care is more important, as long as I can afford the difference. Which plans will let me pick my own doc?"

"Both of the regular (indemnity) insurance plans leave the choice of doctor entirely up to you. The third plan is a preferred provider organization—a PPO. That could be a good choice for you if your doctor is a member. Check the list of doctors in that plan. If your doctor is there and you decide to go with that plan, call his office before you actually sign up, just to make sure he's still a member."

"Will the Schedule of Benefits tell me where I can get medications with each plan? One of my friends has to get all his medicine through the mail. He had a lot of problems with his insulin last summer because it wasn't kept under refrigeration. Those mail trucks get pretty hot. I'd like a plan that lets me go right to the pharmacy."

"Well, that's one thing you don't have to worry about, Mike. All of the plans we're offering this year let you get your medicines from a local pharmacy. But some of them only work with certain pharmacies. So you may want to check that out when you're reviewing the plans."

"OK, I'll put that on my list, too. It sounds like I've got what I need to compare the plans and make a decision. Thanks for the help, Carrie."

"You're welcome, Mike. But there are a few more things you should keep in mind. Read the policies carefully to see if there are any 'exclusions'—things they don't cover— that are important to you. No health insurance plan covers everything and most only pay a part of the cost of things that *are* covered. But before choosing a plan, be sure that it covers the things that are important to you."

"Thanks for the warning. I made a list of the things I'm looking for and that's what I'm going to use to check out these plans before I make my choice." (See Insurance Benefits Shopping List, page 165.)

"Good for you, Mike. And when you've made your choice, fill out the application completely and accurately. Don't try to hide the fact that you have diabetes. That would probably back-fire on you later and your claims could be denied because you withheld information."

Mike could see that his work was cut out for him. Comparing the costs and benefits of each of the plans would take quite a bit of time. But when open enrollment came around, he would be ready to make a good choice.

Insurance Benefits Shopping List*

Office or Clinic Services

- *Doctor Visits:* Most outpatient plans cover doctor fees, but if you use other providers (nurse, dietitian, podiatrist, etc.), check to see if they are covered.

- *Lab Work:* Most "medically necessary" tests ordered by a doctor are covered. You may want to check to see if the following tests are covered: angiography, fluorophotometric tests and other eye and retina tests, and kidney function tests.

- *Diabetes Education*: Few policies cover education separately. Look for coverage as part of covered physician care.

- *Foot Care:* Look for "medically necessary" care of the feet and nails as well as treatment for structural abnormalities or other conditions related to diabetes.

- *Annual Eye Exam:* Look for coverage to detect early signs of diabetes-related eye problems, especially retinopathy.

*No insurance plan covers everything. Decide which services are important to you, then "shop" the available plans to find the one that meets your needs at the best cost.

Medication

- *Prescription drugs* are often covered but check for coverage on insulin (nonprescription).

Equipment and Supplies

- *Equipment:* Meters, insulin pumps, and therapeutic shoes may or may not be covered. Check specifically for items you use. Even when these items are covered, insurance companies may require extra documentation of medical necessity before granting approval.

- *Supplies:* If supplies (syringes, test strips, foot care supplies, pump supplies, etc.) are covered, check for limits such as 2 syringes a day or a given number of test strips per month, and compare the limits to your needs.

If you think
taking care of
diabetes is
expensive,
try the cost
of NOT taking
care of it.

15

Summer Camp: Hormones, Adolescence, and Diabetes

Hello, Mudda. Hello, Fodda,
Here I am at Camp Granada!
—Allen Sherman

The sun was shining so Mike decided to put the top down on his car for the drive to the doctor's office. It had been a while since he'd been there. His visits were less frequent now that his diabetes was in good control. He thought of them like the oil changes on his car. Every 3,000 miles he had the oil changed and the car greased. The car dealer called it "preventive maintenance:" a check to make sure that everything was running smoothly, a way to prevent a major breakdown. Mike wouldn't skip an oil change just because his car was running well. And he wouldn't skip his doctor visits because his diabetes was in good control either. His body was at least as important as his precious convertible. As Arnold Palmer said, "It pays to keep up the old equipment."

He pulled up to the office, parked his car, and walked into the waiting room. He nodded to the receptionist and scanned the magazine rack. He liked the selection of up-to-date magazines they kept in the waiting room. What a difference from some of the other medical offices he'd been in. He settled down with an article on places to go for a summer vacation.

He *did* have some time off coming. Maybe he could get away for a couple of weeks later in the summer. The sun-splashed beaches in the magazine looked inviting. But just as he was getting into the article, the nurse called his name and said that the doctor was ready to see him.

"Darn," Mike thought to himself. "Why is it that doctors who keep you waiting forever have old boring magazines and the ones who see you on time have great reading material?" He reluctantly put down the magazine and went into the examining room. The nurse weighed him and checked his blood pressure. Then the doctor came in.

"Hi, Mike," the doctor said. "How are you doing?"

"Fine, Doc," Mike replied. "No bad low blood sugar reactions since the last time I saw you. And my finger stick blood sugars are generally where we want them to be."

The doctor looked through the log book and said, "Mike, there's been such an improvement since the first time I saw you. Your finger sticks are mostly in the normal range. And look at your most recent lab sheet. Your glycosylated hemoglobin is only a half percent above normal. You're doing a great job."

"Thanks, Doc. But, you know, the best part's not the numbers. It's the fact that my diabetes is finally on the back burner. I feel good, and I'm not running myself ragged to do it."

"That's great, Mike. You know, you've been on my mind lately. Diabetes Summer Camp is held during the last two weeks in July. When I heard that we needed a few more counselors, I thought of you. You've had a lot of personal experience learning how to control your diabetes. And you know what it feels like to be a teenager with diabetes. You could be a big help. Are you interested?"

"I was planning to take a vacation, Doc, but I was thinking more along the lines of becoming a serious full-time beach bum for a while."

"Well, then, this would be perfect. The camp is right next to a small lake. It's not exactly the ocean, but it's big enough for swimming. In fact, we'll even let you use one of the high-powered camp canoes if you like. All kidding aside, Mike, I wish you'd give it some serious thought. You'd be a great role model for the kids, and I think you'd get a lot of enjoyment out of doing it."

"Sure, Doc. I'll do it," Mike said. "I can always go to the beach for a long weekend later. Where can I get all the details?"

The doctor pulled an envelope out of the desk drawer and handed it to him. "Mike" was written across the front.

"Why do I feel like a mouse that just nibbled on the wrong piece of cheese?" Mike laughed.

A few weeks later, Mike pulled through the gates of the camp and parked his car. The camp was nestled in the woods along a beautiful lake, just like the doctor said it was. But in spite of the peaceful setting, things were pretty hectic. Parents were dropping off children. Kids of all sizes were running in every direction.

"What chaos," Mike thought. There were about 100 of them. The responsibility was awesome.

Things quieted down after the parents left. The campers, counselors, and staff members all started to settle in. After he'd found the teen cabin that was to be his home for the next two weeks, Mike stowed his gear and headed over to the dining hall for supper. When he walked through the door, the first thing he saw was a teenage girl lying unconscious on the floor. One of the camp nurses was kneeling next to her, giving her a shot of glucagon. Mike glanced back at the scene several times as he filled up his tray. Within a few minutes, she started to wake up. Someone gave her a glass of apple juice and she drank it. Finally, she stood up, walked to a table and sat down.

Mike was surprised. The whole episode had caused very little excitement. The treatment was quick and effective. And the campers seemed to take it in stride. Mike carried his tray over to the table where he saw his doctor already eating.

"Did you see that?" Mike asked. "I'm really impressed at how smoothly the staff handled that."

"Have a seat, Mike," the doctor said. "That's one of the big advantages of camp. Outside of diabetes camp, a low blood sugar reaction like that one could cause real chaos. People in other settings aren't usually so well prepared. I'm sure it was still embarrassing for her, but not like it would have been elsewhere."

Mike knew exactly what the doctor was talking about. He'd had a very low blood sugar reaction at his desk last year and someone called the paramedics. He was the talk of the office for the rest of the day. What an embarrassing situation. But here at camp, the severe reaction was taken in stride because everyone knew what was happening and how to handle it. It wasn't such a big deal.

"You know, Mike, this is the first time some of these kids have met someone else with diabetes, except maybe an older aunt or uncle with Type II diabetes. It's great for them to meet each other. It gives them a chance to talk about what it's like to be a kid with diabetes, to give each other support, and to not feel different for a change.

"And for some of them, it's also the first time they've been away from their parents. Camp is a safe place to prove to themselves and their parents that they can take care of themselves and their diabetes."

There was a campfire after supper and the rest of the evening went smoothly. But the next day, as Mike was entering the dining hall for supper, he saw the same girl down on the ground. It was like an instant replay. The same nurse was even giving her glucagon.

This time when she came to, Mike and the doctor asked her to join them at their table. Everyone introduced themselves. The girl's name was Sarah. She was 16 and at camp for the first time. She'd had diabetes for five years.

"I'm sorry to see you having so many insulin reactions," the doctor told Sarah. "I've seen that happen before though. In fact, there are almost always some kids who have extra reactions their first few days at camp. There's so much going on here. Most campers get a lot more exercise than they do at home. So they need less insulin. It usually takes a few days to find the right dose.

"But," he went on, "I'm not sure that's what's happening with you, Sarah. You don't seem to be doing a lot with the other kids. Why is that?"

"Oh, I don't know. Maybe because I really don't know anyone here," she answered.

Just then the cook arrived with the food. There was plenty of it and it smelled great. She set down platters of grilled chicken and baked potatoes and followed up with large bowls of carrots and zucchini. The salad looked fresh and colorful. Everyone was hungry after a long day of swimming and hiking. The noisy dining hall quieted down as everyone dug in and began to eat.

Well, almost everyone. Mike noticed that Sarah wasn't really eating. She'd put very little food on her plate and was barely picking at it.

"Aren't you hungry, Sarah?" Mike asked.

"No, not really." She pushed the carrots around her plate one more time.

"Gee, why are you eating so little, Sarah? I'm usually so hungry I could eat chairs after I have a bad reaction," said one of the other girls at the table.

"If you must know, I'm on a diet. I'm trying to lose some weight."

The word "diet" was like a light going on in the doctor's head. He remembered seeing Sarah just pick up a diet soda pop at the snack table that afternoon. She was having those severe reactions because she wasn't eating enough.

The doctor knew that trying to work on this problem would involve dealing with Sarah's body image. Feeling good about your own body is a big issue for teenagers. "But teenagers aren't the only ones," the doctor thought. "Considering the number of adults on weight loss diets, it's obviously a problem for some people all through their lives." He searched for the right words to discuss the problem with Sarah.

"It sounds like dieting has thrown your insulin and food intake out of balance, Sarah. The way to stop those reactions is to get them matched up again. And you know, having to eat extra food every day to treat insulin reactions makes it hard to stick with a food plan to lose weight."

"I know," she answered. "But I feel like such a dweeb sometimes because of my diabetes. I think if I could lose a few pounds and look better, maybe I'd get along better. It's not fair. Other girls at school skip meals to stay thin and nothing happens to them."

"You're right, it isn't fair," the doctor answered. "Still, I'd like to tell you something you're going to have trouble believing right now: A few pounds one way or the other won't make that much difference in how the other kids treat you. It'd be great if it was that easy. I'll bet if we could get people talking about it, you'd find out that there are plenty of thin and fit kids here who sometimes feel out of place, too. Try not to expect too much out of losing a few pounds.

"But if you like, I can look at your meal plan and insulin dose to help you figure out how to get more fit. Still, I have to warn you, Sarah. Eating like a bird won't get you where you want to be. You need to think about getting some exercise, too."

"OK, Doctor. I guess I can give it a try," Sarah answered.

The doctor had seen people try to lose weight by cutting back on their insulin and allowing their blood sugars to go high. But they paid a high price for losing a few pounds that way. Besides losing fat, they also lost muscle, diabetes control, and, if they ended up in diabetic ketoacidosis, sometimes a lot more.

He wondered why some people worried so much about their weight, to the point that they endangered their health. He wanted his patients to feel good and be as healthy as possible. That involved a lot more than just getting on a scale and weighing themselves everyday.

"Obviously this isn't a problem I can solve single-handedly," he thought as he talked with Sarah for a few more minutes. But the meal was ending and it was time to get ready for the evening campfire. Tomorrow was another day and maybe in the coming week he'd be able to discuss it with her some more, maybe even involve her parents. Maybe not.

On Tuesday morning Mike was scheduled to help the diabetes educator man the blood-testing station before breakfast. Several campers had already come and gone when Lucy, one of the junior counselors, arrived. When she looked up after completing the test, her eyes were filled with tears.

"What's wrong, Lucy?" the educator asked. "Is there anything I can do to help?"

"I don't think so, Kate. It's hopeless. No matter what I do anymore, my blood sugars are a mess. And my folks are really upset. They think I'm eating sweets or something. But I'm really not. I'm doing the same things I've always done, but instead of my sugars being where they should be, they're all over the place. I thought they'd get better up here because of all the exercise, but it's just the same."

"That must be so frustrating for you, Lucy. Do you mind my asking how old you are?"

"Almost 14," she offered.

"I thought so. Lucy, have you heard about how your hormones go on the march when you get to be a teenager?"

"Yeah, sure. I know all about puberty, periods, and pimples!"

"Well, the same hormones that do all those things for you and complicate your life can also make it really difficult to control your diabetes. I think that may be at least part of the reason for those high blood sugars that are upsetting you and your parents so much. Almost every teenager with diabetes has the same problem, to one extent or another. I have an article about this that you might like to read and show to your parents. It won't help your blood sugars, but it may take some of the pressure and frustration off you and your folks. And talk to your doctor about this the next time you see her. She may want to change your target blood sugar levels until your hormones level off."

"Thanks, Kate. Can I get the article from you this afternoon?"

"Sure, Lucy. Come over to my office in the community hall after lunch."

After the last of the campers finished their blood tests and went in to the dining hall, Mike turned to the educator. "Where were you when I was a teenager, Kate? There were times when a little information like that sure could have smoothed things out for me. You did a nice thing for Lucy."

"Thanks, Mike. That's one of the big enjoyments I get out of my job. Sometimes you get to do a nice thing. Are you enjoying being a counselor?"

"To be honest, I had my doubts at first," he replied. "But now I'm really getting to like it. Let's go get some breakfast."

The next day Mike was on the soccer field. It was the Reds against the Blues. Mike was on the Blue team. He'd played soccer in high school and it was great to be playing again. The teams were evenly matched so possession of the ball turned over from one team to the other very quickly. Mike was running up and down the field constantly. It was demanding. But he was in shape and able to do it. Then he noticed that one of his teammates wasn't doing as well.

His name was Tom. He was 15 and the whole team knew how much he wanted to play on his school's varsity soccer team. Mike had to admit he was determined. He worked out everyday trying to build himself up. But he was a skinny kid and didn't seem to have much strength or staying power. And he was always thirsty. At first, Mike thought the thirst was being caused by the summer sun, but then he realized no one else was drinking as much as Tom. Mike was concerned and suggested that the boy see the doctor at morning sick call.

Tom reported to sick call right after breakfast the next morning. The nurse measured his height and weight and did a finger stick blood sugar. It was 310. Even though Tom thought that the blood sugar was high because he'd just eaten breakfast, the doctor was suspicious. He had the nurse check Tom's urine for ketones. The test was positive. There were ketones in Tom's urine.

"Tom," the doctor said, "Mike has told me how much you love soccer. He said that you're planning to try out for your school's team in the fall."

"That's right, Doc."

"But he also tells me you have trouble keeping up with the other boys."

"I do my best, Doc. I try hard and I exercise every day. I'll get better. The coach says all I really need is desire, and I've sure got that."

"That kind of motivation is great to see, Tom. But I think your diabetes may be holding you back from reaching your goal. Look at these height and weight tables for your age. According to the chart your doctor sent along, it looks like you haven't been growing as much as you should be lately. You used to be relatively big for your age. Now, suddenly, you're on the small side."

"But Doc, how can that be? My father's tall and all my brothers are big, too. Won't I be big like them?"

"Not if your diabetes stays out of control."

"What do you mean?"

"Tom, when your diabetes is way out of control, your body can't grow and develop as it should. Right now you're spilling ketones in the urine and your blood sugar is quite high. When that's going on, calories from the food you eat end up in your urine instead of being used as building blocks for your body.

"You're a teenager. About now you should be having what we call a growth spurt—a time when you move pretty rapidly from your kid-size body into your adult size. But that won't happen with your diabetes out of control. You'll only grow up to your full potential size if your blood sugars stay in better control. If you don't keep them under control, you may wind up shorter and with less muscle than you should have."

"But, Doc, I exercise all the time. Won't that build up my body?"

"Only if your diabetes is pretty well managed, Tom. When you build a house, you have to put it on a solid foundation. If the foundation is weak, the entire house will crumble. It's the same thing with your body. Eating healthy foods and maintaining good control of your diabetes is the foundation you need to lay down before you can build up your body with exercise. Without that foundation, all the exercise in the world won't give you the strength and endurance you want. When diabetes is out of control, your body just can't build muscle mass."

"I never knew that. Okay, Doc, what do I need to do?"

"First, I'm going to increase your insulin to get rid of those ketones. Then let's start getting some blood sugar readings. By the time you go home, things should be looking a lot better."

As soon as the ketones cleared, Tom noticed how much more energy he had. And he was playing better. His weight was even up a few pounds by the end of the week. He'd been trying to gain weight all spring without success. Now that he understood what was going on, he could see that he needed to make diabetes control part of his training program.

At the soccer game on Friday, Tom waved at Mike. "Thanks for sending me in to see the doctor, Mike. I think it's going to make a big difference."

"That's great news. You're looking a lot stronger out there, Tom. Let me know when you make the team. I'd love to come and watch you play."

After the game, Mike walked back toward his cabin. He wished that things were going as well for Brian as they were for Tom. Brian was one of the boys in his cabin. He was 12 years old and an only child. Mike had watched the boy and overheard some talk in the cabin that worried him. It seemed that Brian used his diabetes to get what he wanted from his parents. He'd found out that if he made his blood sugars go out of control, he could get just about anything he wanted.

He bragged to the other boys about how he could skip a meal to bring on a bad reaction or eat a lot of sweets or even squirt his insulin down the drain to send his blood sugar so high it didn't even register on his meter.

Mike remembered doing some pretty outrageous things himself when he was about Brian's age. Life had seemed so unfair. But his parents had been strict about certain things. They even "kept him company" while he took his shots for a while. Things had eventually straightened out. He hoped that Brian would be as lucky.

Mike got busy after supper preparing for the hiking contest that was on the schedule for the next morning. Each hiker would get a whistle, a map of the course through the woods that he'd laid out, and a compass. The first one to complete the course would get the grand prize—no kitchen duty for two days.

Saturday morning dawned warm and beautiful. Seventeen hikers set off down the course. Mike was waiting at the finish line when the first hiker returned to camp at mid-morning. It was Brian. Mike was still shaking the young man's hand when one of the other counselors came down the trail out of the woods.

"Brian, I'm sorry," she said, "but I saw you leave the course and take a short cut. I won't say anything in front of the others, but I have to disqualify you."

Brian glared at her and Mike. "It's just a stupid kid's game anyway. I could've won if I'd wanted to. You'll be sorry you treated me like this." Brian stomped off in the direction of the cabin and remained out of sight for the rest of the afternoon.

Later, he ignored Mike's invitation to sit with him at dinner. Instead, he walked to an empty table near the door to the kitchen. The next time Mike saw Brian, the boy was sitting on a rock at the far edge of the evening campfire gathering. He walked over and stood next to him.

"Didn't see you eating much dinner, Brian."

"So what," the boy replied.

"Planning on having a reaction here pretty soon?"

"Soon enough."

"Brian, you're not at home. You're at camp. There are rules here. If you don't follow them, there are consequences. At home, taking out your anger by not eating may shake your parents up and cause a lot of excitement. Around here all it'll get you is a few dirty looks and a one-way ticket back home. I'd hate to see that happen. You've got a great sense of humor. You brought the house down at lunch yesterday. But your behavior cut you off from all the fun today. Take some advice from somebody who's been there. Stop using your diabetes like a club on the people around you. It's dangerous. And it doesn't do much for your popularity either."

The next morning Mike went over to sick call to talk to the doctor about Brian.

"I'm not sure I did the right thing, Doc."

"Oh, I think you did just fine, Mike. You showed Brian that you care and maybe what you said will make him reconsider what he's doing. Being a teenager is a tough job, even if you don't have diabetes. There's so much change. Your body changes into somebody else's. Your hormones go on a rampage. You try to figure out who you are and how you fit in with the rest of the world. A lot of youngsters with diabetes use their condition to act out all that turmoil. In some ways, it's just another situation they might use to figure out who they are. It's something like wearing trendy clothing and extreme hair styles, listening to loud music, or having friends who drive their parents crazy. But it's different from those things, too, because it can be a lot more dangerous.

"I try to encourage my teenage patients to find safer ways to establish their identity than skipping meals or insulin shots or writing down blood sugar tests they never did. But those things still happen sometimes. Parents need to recognize, without laying blame, the possibility that this kind of behavior is going to come up sometimes. But they still need to set some guidelines. When that happens, both the kids and the parents will probably survive adolescence."

"I remember the doctor I used to see when I was a teenager," Mike said. "When I was doing this kind of stuff, he told me, 'You've got to be a teenager, Mike, but try to leave your diabetes out of it as much as you can. Do it the way your friends do. Dye your hair blue if you want, but, for goodness sake, don't skip your insulin!'"

"He sounds like a wise man. But, Mike, do me a favor. Don't spread that advice around too much up here. I don't want to have to explain a lot of blue hair and pierced noses to irate parents on the last day of camp."

"OK, Doc. I'll try to keep it to myself. By the way, thanks for luring me up here. It's been great."

Being a teenager
is hard.

Having diabetes
makes it harder.

16

What Can We Learn from the Black Box? Research

Sweet dreams and flying machines
in pieces on the ground.
—James Taylor

"You know, Doc, my sister is worried she might get diabetes like I did."

"It's not like the flu, Mike. She can't catch it from you."

"Oh, she knows that, but she's worried because we have diabetes in the family. She thinks she'll get it too. She even borrows my meter once in a while to test her blood sugar, to make sure she doesn't have it yet."

"That's understandable. Fear of developing diabetes is a common worry in the families of people who already have it. Brothers and sisters worry they'll get the disease. Parents worry their other children will develop diabetes. And the people who actually have it worry about whether they should have children themselves for fear their kids may end up with diabetes, too. So your sister's not alone in her concerns.

"But tell her there's a better test than a finger-stick blood sugar to let her know what's going on."

"What test is that?"

"It's called an *islet-cell antibody test.*"

"How does it work?"

"Well, Mike, we've talked about the fact that you developed Type I diabetes when the beta cells in your pancreas were destroyed. We know the body's own immune system is involved in this somehow. But we don't know yet exactly what happens.

"When the immune system is destroying the beta cells, something called the islet-cell antibody shows up in the bloodstream. The antibody is there long before the blood sugar level shoots up. That's one of the reasons it's a better test for your sister than a finger-stick blood sugar. The presence of the islet-cell antibody in the bloodstream is an early sign that Type I diabetes has begun to develop. There are other antibodies that can also be used to predict diabetes. And research is being done in order to understand them better. But the islet-cell antibody test is the first test of its kind to be made widely available."

"So this test can tell years in advance if someone is likely to get diabetes?"

"Right."

"That sounds like a really depressing piece of news to me. What possible good can come out of knowing for years that you're going to end up taking insulin and testing your blood someday?"

"I'm sure it sounds that way at first, Mike. But it's actually critical information. It's important, not only to the person who has the test done, but also to everyone who might develop Type I diabetes in the future. That islet-cell antibody test is like the flight data recorder on a commercial airliner—that thing they call the 'Black Box.'"

"Doc, you sure have a lot of stories about flying and airplanes. Are you a frustrated pilot?"

"Well, now you know my secret, Mike. But let me explain what I mean. When an airplane goes down, investigators show up at the crash site searching for clues. Their first job is to find the Black Box. Everything that happened in the final moments of the flight is recorded in that box. They use that information to reconstruct the flight and pinpoint the exact cause of the crash. Their goal is to prevent future accidents."

"So you're saying the beta cells of a person developing Type I diabetes are like a plane headed for a crash?"

"Yes, in a way, they are. And we hope that by improving our knowledge of how diabetes develops, we'll be able to figure out how to prevent it in the future."

"Now that's information that would really interest my sister. How can screening for the islet-cell antibody help?"

"Before the test for the antibody was available, researchers were limited to examining the aftermath of the 'crash.' It was like trying to figure out what had caused a plane to crash in the days before the Black Box. Without a Black Box, the only sources of available information were the pieces on the ground. Specific information about what happened just before the crash wasn't available until the development of the Black Box. It provides a wealth of information, including the airplane's final course, attitude, and speed. Knowing what occurred just before the crash helps the investigators figure out how to prevent the same thing from happening again.

"By monitoring changes in islet-cell antibodies and blood insulin levels, diabetes researchers have begun to get an accurate picture of the events that lead up to the 'crash' of the beta cell. Now they're no longer working with just the pieces on the ground. They can identify people who will develop Type I diabetes years before their symptoms start—even before their blood sugars begin to rise. Researchers can then follow these people to find out what goes wrong and to figure out a way to prevent the crash of the beta cell.

"Islet-cell antibody testing has already given us a very important piece of information—namely, that Type I diabetes develops over a period of several years."

"Not for me, Doc! My diabetes came on very suddenly. One day I was perfectly fine, doing everything I'd always done. Then, almost overnight, I was drinking everything I could get my hands on and urinating constantly—eating everything in sight but losing weight. That change only took a couple of weeks, not years."

"I know what you're saying, Mike. I was actually taught in medical school that Type I diabetes develops very rapidly. But that's not true. Although the *symptoms* come on suddenly, the disease itself actually develops over a long period of time. Some people have gone as long as ten years from the time they were first found to have islet-cell antibodies until they developed diabetes. They felt fine until right before the diagnosis was made, but their ability to make insulin had been falling with every year that passed."

"How could they have normal blood sugars and feel fine if they were making less insulin?"

"We think it's because the body has a relatively huge supply of beta cells, compared with the need for insulin. Researchers say that as many as 90 percent of the cells have to be destroyed before the blood sugar begins to rise.

To look at it another way, once the blood sugar is abnormal, almost all the beta cells have already been destroyed."

"So you think my sister should get the islet-cell antibody test?"*

"Yes, Mike, I do. Using information from enough people like your sister—people who have brothers, sisters, parents, or children with Type I diabetes—researchers may be able to understand the whole process of beta cell destruction and eventually come up with a way to prevent it."

---

* Various research centers, including the Joslin Diabetes Center in Boston, Massachusetts, can perform islet-cell antibody testing for relatives of persons throughout the country with Type I diabetes. Call the Joslin Clinic at (617) 732-2546 for more information.

Research done now might stop diabetes in the future.

17

Is There a History of Death in your Family? Complications

Now the darkness only stays a nighttime.
In the morning it will fade away.
Daylight is good at arriving at the right time.
—George Harrison

It was Sunday evening. The young man was walking along the beach to watch the sunset. A few lazy clouds hung motionless near the horizon as the yellow glare of the afternoon sun softened to a pink and golden glow.

A familiar form shifted position on the rocks near the water's edge. It was Mike's doctor. He sat gazing silently across the bay at the setting sun.

"Hi, Doc."

"Hi, Mike."

"What are you up to?" Mike asked.

"Oh, just sitting here thinking."

"About what?"

"Life, actually. Sometimes I come down here to think about life. It helps me keep things in perspective."

"Perspective?"

"Well, I see a lot of people in the course of a day—often when things aren't going too well for them. They're sick and they're worried or scared. Or someone they care about is sick. And sometimes they share their deepest thoughts and concerns with me. I get to see a side of life that most people don't."

"I imagine that's pretty hard to take sometimes."

"Yes, it is. But on the other hand, it's taught me a lot."

"Like what?" Mike asked.

"Like how people respond when life throws them a curve. I've seen people respond in very different ways."

"I can tell you how I responded to being told I had diabetes.

I got depressed. Actually I was real scared at first. And then I got angry. Since then I've been mostly frustrated. It's been a lot better since I've learned to take care of myself, but it still gets me down. Especially when I think about the long-term picture."

"I understand," the doctor replied. "A lot of my patients have told me similar stories. But what's really amazing to me—what really makes me think about my own outlook on life—is how some of my patients have actually turned that situation around to their own advantage."

"Give me a break, Doc. You can't tell me there's anything good about having diabetes. It's a royal pain."

"Yeah, there's no doubt diabetes is a hard hand to play. But some people seem to play it very well. They wind up eating better and getting more exercise than they did before. They live each day to the fullest. It's as if, for some people, the diabetes is a constant reminder to push ahead and live well. And then there are others who seem to see diabetes as something that holds them back."

"It's a good point, Doc. Nobody's life is perfect. You do have to play the hand you're dealt. After all, it's the only one you have. But every time I pick up a book about diabetes, I'm reminded of those long-term complications. I feel like the clock is running, and it's just a matter of time until the complications start. I ask myself, 'When will my eyes start to bother me? How long will my kidneys last?' Some of the numbers are frightening."

"This is something I discuss with my patients quite often," the doctor said. "It's an area where perspective is really important. To put your concern about complications in perspective, we need to talk about two things: one is the way diabetes care has changed in the last few years and the other is the history of death in your family."

"What do you mean?"

"Well, if you go back as far as 1921, before insulin was available, a diagnosis of Type I diabetes meant death in six months to two years. But then insulin became available and the book had to be rewritten. With insulin, people survived. In fact, they survived long enough to develop the complications we worry so much about today.

"Those frightening numbers you talked about earlier—the ones quoted as the chance you'll develop a certain complication in a given number of years—were developed between the 1920's and the 1980's, a period when the standard of diabetes management was very different from what it is today.

"Now, patients are actively involved in their own care and we have a lot of technical advances at our fingertips. We can achieve much better blood sugar control than was possible at the time those statistics were compiled. Together with control of cholesterol and blood pressure, better blood sugar control can help prevent the tissue damage that leads to diabetes complications. I think we're going to rewrite the book again in the 1990's."

"That makes sense to me, Doc. But what do you mean, 'The history of death in my family?' Everyone has a history of death in their family."

"Exactly!" the doctor answered. "Everyone is going to die. All of your ancestors have done it, and you're going to do it, too. And the same would be true even if you didn't have diabetes. Everyone will die of something. And all of us—whether we have diabetes or not—have some tendency to develop health problems as we get older. How much of a tendency—or 'risk'—we have varies.

"One of the things that affects our risk for health problems is how good a job we did of picking our parents—in other words, our genetic tendencies. If we picked parents who made the mistake of dying at a young age of heart disease, our risk is greater than if we'd been smart enough to pick parents who lived to a ripe old age.

"Of course, I'm kidding you a bit, but the point is this: We all have some degree of risk for developing health problems as we go through life. A portion of that risk can't be controlled. Diabetes adds to the risk, but it doesn't make health problems a certainty.

"On the other hand, there ARE things that influence risk that we DO have control over: eating well, staying physically active, avoiding smoking and substance abuse, and keeping blood pressure and blood sugar under control. These are things we can do to minimize whatever risk we have inherited from our parents or acquired through developing diabetes."

"I think you're right," replied the young man. "I guess whether we have diabetes or not, we only have so much tread on our tires. And it's a matter of trying to get the most mileage possible out of the tread we've got."

"Now you're telling stories, too," the doctor observed. "Think you've spent too much time with us?"

"Not really," Mike replied. "Sometimes the stories help me see things more clearly. They get the point across and make the facts easier to remember."

The doctor motioned to Mike and they walked back up the beach. "It's too late now to go back and pick different parents, Mike. And you can't get rid of your diabetes just yet either—although you may see that happen in your lifetime. So, as the old philosopher says, 'A wise man accepts what he can't change.'

"But the things you CAN change—the things you DO have control over—what you eat, how much you exercise, how well you control your blood sugar, blood pressure and cholesterol, whether or not you smoke, whether or not you wear your seat belt when you get in the car, and so on, are well worth the effort. They can make a difference. And that's just as true for people who don't have diabetes as it is for those who do.

"Remember your family not only has a history of death, it also has a history of LIFE!

"Go out and live it well!"

There is hope.

You have control!

Index